FRANNY CHRISTMAS.

COMMUNITY HEALTH
AND
SOCIAL SERVICES

Fourth Edition

Brian Meredith Davies
MD (London), FFCM, DPH

Formerly Director of Social Services, City of Liverpool
Lecturer in Clinical (Preventive) Paediatrics, University of Liverpool

GW00372809

HODDER AND STOUGHTON
LONDON SYDNEY AUCKLAND TORONTO

MODERN NURSING SERIES

General Editor
SUSAN E NORMAN, SRN, DN CERT, RNT
Senior Tutor, Nightingale School, West Lambeth Health Authority

Consultant Editor
A J HARDING RAINS, MS, FRCS,
Regional Dean, British Postgraduate Medical Federation; formerly Professor of Surgery, Charing Cross Hospital Medical School, University of London; Honorary Consultant Surgeon, Charing Cross Hospital; Honorary Consultant Surgeon to the Army

---

British Library Cataloguing in Publication Data

Davies, Brian Meredith
   Community health and social services.—4th ed.
   1. Community health services—Great Britain
   2. Public welfare—Great Britain
   3. Nursing—Great Britain
   I. Title
   361'.941'024613   HV245

   ISBN 0 340 32387 6

First published as *Preventive Medicine for Nurses and Social Workers*, 1965
Second edition 1972, reprinted with extensive revisions, 1975
Third edition 1977, reprinted with extensive revisions, 1980
Fourth edition 1984, third impression 1986

Typeset in 10/11 pt Times by Macmillan India Ltd, Bangalore.

Printed in Great Britain for
Hodder and Stoughton Educational,
a division of Hodder and Stoughton Ltd.,
Mill Road, Dunton Green, Sevenoaks, Kent TN13 2YD,
by Richard Clay Ltd, Bungay, Suffolk

Editors' Foreword

This well established series of books reflects contemporary nursing and health care practice. It is used by a wide range of nursing, medical and ancillary professions and encompasses titles suitable for different levels of experience from those in training to those who have qualified.

Members of the nursing professions need to be highly informed and to keep critically abreast of demanding changes in attitudes and technology. The series therefore continues to grow with new titles being added to the list and existing titles being updated regularly. Its aim is to promote sound understanding by presenting essential facts clearly and concisely. We hope this will lead to nursing care of the highest standard.

Preface

Since the last edition 5 years ago there have been many changes and advances in preventive medicine, in the National Health Service and in the personal social services. These changes are fully described in this edition and include the latest alterations to the organisation of the health services introduced in 1982 in an attempt to reduce bureaucracy and to increase the efficiency of the services. There are now only 2 tiers of health authorities—the 14 Regional Health Authorities, and the new 192 District Health Authorities in England and 9 in Wales.

This edition follows the format of earlier ones and is divided into 2 parts covering (a) the community health services and (b) the personal social services. The interdependence of both is becoming more evident as the recession deepens making more vulnerable many of the elderly, mentally disabled, physically disabled and children in need. It is becoming clear that, in future, more and more people who fall ill or who are chronically handicapped or elderly will have to be cared for at home. The quality of care they receive will depend upon the understanding by nurses working in hospitals and in the community of the range of services and help which is available. At these times of cutbacks and recession it is equally important for these vulnerable groups themselves to know what services are available in the community and to use them sensibly. Too often in recent years a contributory factor in serious cases of neglect has been the ignorance of the individual, the family or neighbours to know what help they can obtain (whether financial help or aid in kind) and how to go about getting it. It is never easy to spread this type of information to the general public but one of the more effective ways is for professionals in hospital to do this in the course of their work.

It is hoped that this short book will provide a simple and readable introduction to the community health and personal social services. It should help both the nurse in training and the trained nurse to keep up to date in this important field.

All the indicators described in Chapter 2 to measure health have been revised. Other changes include full descriptions of the important new screening tests to discover (1) neural tube defects in the foetus in sufficient time to terminate the pregnancy, and (2) hypothyroidism in the new born infant, so enabling early treatment; this treatment is easy to carry out and safe and will not affect the eventual intelligence of the child.

The Education Act 1981 which introduced some of the more important features of the Warnock Report dealing with the education of handicapped children and those with special needs is fully explained.

Recent years have also seen many changes in the field of mental health culminating in the Mental Health Act 1983 which is now operational and which introduced important changes aimed at increasing the safeguards for mentally ill persons who have to be compulsorily detained in hospital. These are fully described. Reference is made to the Mental Health Act Commission and to the extended powers and use to be made of the Mental Health Review Tribunals in the future.

The strains placed upon both the health and personal social services by the increasing proportions of the elderly population over the age of 85 years are already becoming apparent. From the present day figure of just under 1 in 100 of the total population, the over 85 year olds will rise to 1 in 65 by the year 2000. As so many of the worst health and social problems are found in this very vulnerable age group, it is obvious that effective community care for them is essential. Chapter 16 describes the latest services for this small but very important group of elderly persons with special emphasis on preventive health measures. It cannot be too strongly emphasised that many of the crises in the very old could be avoided or markedly reduced *if only the right steps are taken earlier in retirement.* It is therefore becoming important for the nurse to understand how people can be helped by sound preparation for their retirement.

Once again I would like to thank my wife for all her patient help with the typing of the script and correction of the proofs and for the compilation of the index as well as for her constant encouragement.

1984   Brian Meredith Davies

Contents

1
The Structure of the Reorganized Health Services

Before discussing the various parts of the community health services and the ways in which disease is prevented, it is important that the structure of the health services is fully understood.

The National Health Service in the United Kingdom was introduced in 1948 and was completely reorganized in 1974 and 1982. It is an essential part of a much wider system of social security in which the whole state makes compulsory provision for various inevitable happenings in life, including the prevention of disease and the treatment of illness. The National Health Service is a comprehensive health service covering the whole country and its benefits and services are available to everyone. There is no contracting out of the service and it is financed centrally from both Exchequer general taxation and specific levies paid within National Insurance contributions.

Function of the Secretary of State for Social Services

The Secretary of State for Social Services has full overall responsibility for the health and social services and is responsible directly to Parliament being a member of the Cabinet. The responsibilities of the Secretary of State for local social services undertaken by local authorities are discussed on pages 170–2.

As regards the health services, the Secretary of State must arrange to provide to an extent which he considers necessary:

1 Accommodation for any services under the National Health Service Acts (clinics, health centres etc.).
2 Hospital accommodation.
3 Medical, dental, nursing and ambulance services.
4 Facilities for the care of expectant and nursing mothers and very young children.
5 Facilities for the prevention of illness and after care of persons suffering from illness. These include vaccination and immunization and a full range of rehabilitation services (including physiotherapy and occupational therapy).
6 Such other services which are required for the diagnosis and treatment of illness (these include full pathological, bacteriological, blood transfusion and mass radiography services).

7 School Health Services (in conjunction with Local Education Authorities).
8 Family Planning Services.

There are a number of *Standing Advisory Committees* (such as the Standing Advisory Committee on Prevention of Disease by Immunization) to which the Secretary of State may refer various specific problems. From time to time, particularly pressing problems occur which need very careful study and the Secretary of State may then arrange for them to be examined in detail by a special *ad hoc* Expert Committee. An example of an Expert Committee was the Court Committee which in 1974–7 studied the future of the child health services (under the chairmanship of Professor Court). Such a committee would collect evidence from various sources, study that evidence and recommend a course of action. It then becomes the responsibility of the Secretary of State for Social Services to assess the report and decide whether to recommend Parliament to implement the changes suggested.

In some instances, the subject to be studied is so important that a Royal Commission may be appointed by Parliament to consider the subject and report. Examples include the Royal Commission on the National Health Service, set up in 1976, which reported in 1979, or the Royal Commission on the law relating to mental illness which was set up in 1955 and whose report in 1958 formed the basis for the change in the law relating to mental illness and handicap by the Mental Health Act 1959.

In addition to these expert committees, the Secretary of State has a large staff of experts to advise him, based at the Department of Health and Social Security in London and locally in various regional offices. These include administrators, doctors, nurses and architects who deal with the detailed administration.

Method of control exercised by the Department of Health and Social Security

The method used to control health services locally varies. Although all day to day administration of the health services is dealt with locally at the District Health Authority level, the Department of Health and Social Security has three methods of controlling overall development.

1 Financial. This is the most important method. All the finance needed for the health services is supplied from the Department of Health and Social Security and covers running costs (*revenue expenditure*) and new buildings (*capital expenditure*).

The Department of Health and Social Security passes regional budgets for each Regional Health Authority which then allocates finances to each individual District Health Authority. In allocating finance to Regional Health Authorities, the Department of Health and Social Security will take regard to special developments which it wishes to encourage. In this way, the Department of Health and Social Security will be able to encourage (by providing the finances necessary) services which it considers urgently need developing.

As regards capital, the Department of Health and Social Security provides finance for hospital building on a 'once and for all' basis and not on any loan basis. All new health centres are financed centrally which ensures a more uniform development of health centres.

2 Advisory. Advice on the development of all aspects of the health services is constantly being issued by the Department of Health and Social Security in the form of memoranda and circulars. In many instances, the advice covers both health and social services. In the publication 'Better services for the mentally ill' issued in 1975, the whole question of the levels of services for the mentally handicapped was discussed and included recommendations of the type and amount of development in hospital and community services and covered the health and social services. In 1974 and in 1980 special circulars were issued on 'non-accidental injury in children'. The circulars advised the way such services should be organized locally and asked for each area to report on its progress in setting up a system of control through Area Review Committees and on the establishment of registers.

3 Planning and policy. The development of an integrated national health service calls for careful planning to ensure that the most urgent needs are met and that services are balanced between the different parts (*i.e.* between hospital, general practice and the community). It is, for instance, no use advocating a reduction in the number of hospital places for a certain group of patients (for example—the mentally ill) if there are not enough community services to help these patients when discharged from hospitals.

In the reorganized health service it is hoped that future planning will be more carefully carried out and will involve local staff of all types through the *Health-Care Planning Teams* (see below). It is hoped that a future long range plan for all the health and social services will be developed each year so that carefully integrated and balanced development will take place. In particular the planning aspect should always consider the *effectiveness of health services* as judged by their benefit to the ordinary people—i.e. are the health services managing to produce better health and less disease and is the health of the majority of the population better?

The Department of Health and Social Security acts as a master planner for the health and social services. By these various methods, the Secretary of State is able to exert an indirect control over the services— strengthening them where they are weakest and constantly encouraging an improvement in standards of care.

Parliamentary control

Because the Secretary of State is answerable to Parliament for the conduct of the health services, it is always open to any member of Parliament to raise any question, however detailed, and this must be answered by the Secretary of State verbally at question time or in writing.

In very serious instances, the Secretary of State can set up an Inquiry which then considers all aspects of the question and reports to the Secretary of State who then presents that report to Parliament. Recent examples have included fires in certain hospitals and allegations about the maltreatment of patients in mental hospitals.

A further method of control was introduced in 1973 by the setting up of a Health Service Commissioner for England and a separate one for Wales (see page 16).

Administration of the National Health Service

The simplest way to understand the functioning of the National Health Service is to look at the plan of its administration (see Fig. 1.1).

It will be seen that since 1982 there are only two types of health authorities, *Regions* and *Districts*. The 14 Regions have remained the same size since 1974 but there are now 192 District Health Authorities, the population of each rarely exceeding 500 000.

It is hoped that the latest reorganization (in 1982) will achieve:

(a) more delegation of responsibility to those in hospitals and in the community health services;

(b) simplification of the professional advisory machinery so that the views of clinical doctors, nurses and other professionals in close contact with patients will be more readily available to the health authorities;

(c) simplification of the planning system which should ensure that regional plans take into account district needs;

(d) strengthening and simplification of hospital management so that staff in hospital carrying out non-clinical functions should be accountable to the hospital administrator rather than to district level managers;

(e) reduction of line management hierarchy.

Secretary of State for Social Services
(advised by officers of the Department of Health
and Social Security — DHSS)

Officers
Central and regional
staff of DHSS

Regional Team of Officers (RTO) ———— *14 Regional Health Authorities (RHAs)*
(each responsible for 8–22 DHAs)

Regional Medical Officer
Regional Nursing Officer
Regional Works Officer
Regional Administrator
Regional Treasurer

Functions include:
Planning and priorities
Appointment of consultants (except in DHAs
with teaching responsibilities)
Allocation of resources between DHAs
Capital building
Postgraduate medical, dental and nurse training
Ambulance duties (may be delegated to DHA)
Blood transfusion service

District Team of Officers (DTO) ——— *192 District Health Authorities (DHAs)*
(each responsible for the functions listed below)

District Medical Officer
District Nursing Officer
District Administrator
District Treasurer
Chairman and Deputy Chairman of
District Medical Committee
(consultant and general practitioner)

Day to day running of all hospital services
Maternity and child welfare
Domiciliary and hospital midwifery
Health visiting
District nursing
Vaccination and immunization
Prevention of disease, care and after-care
Health centres
Appointment of consultants (in DHAs containing
teaching hospitals)

Community Health Councils ———
Represent the patients' interests

Ambulance services (when delegated)

Fig. 1.1   National Health Services—England

Local administration of the health services

Locally, the administration of the health services involves:

(a) Regional Health Authorities (RHAs) and Regional Teams of Officers (RTOs) (see below)
(b) District Health Authorities (DHAs) and District Teams of Officers (DTOs) (see page 9)
(c) Health Care Planning Teams (see page 10)
(d) Community Health Councils (see page 12)

In addition, statutory coordinating committees called *Joint Consultative Committees* are set up to help cooperation between District Health Authorities and neighbouring local authorities responsible for social services, education and housing (see page 11).

Regional Health Authorities (RHAs) and Regional Teams of Officers (RTOs)

Generally the Regional Health Authority (RHA) is responsible for the main planning of health services, for capital building programmes, for postgraduate medical, dental and nurse training and for the allocation of financial resources between the constituent District Health Authorities.

There are 14 RHAs in England and their distribution is shown on Figure 1.2. Each has at least one University providing medical education within its boundaries. The RHA forms part of the chain of responsibility from the Secretary of State to the DHAs.

The main functions of the RHAs include:

1 The development of strategic plans based on the needs identified by the DHAs
2 The allocation of financial resources between its constituent DHAs.
3 Monitoring the performance and policies of each DHA to ensure that they are consistent to the needs of the whole region.
4 The development of a regional plan for specialist services, i.e. deciding the location and provision of the rarer specialities such as chest surgery, radiotherapy, neurosurgery etc.
5 Ensuring with the DHAs that there are adequate medical and dental teaching and research facilities available (this includes postgraduate teaching).
6 Provision of an ambulance service—day to day control may be delegated to larger DHAs with the exception of the large contributions, i.e. London, Birmingham, Liverpool etc.
7 The design and construction of all large capital building developments (i.e. new hospitals). Small capital projects (i.e. health centres) are

Fig. 1.2　National Health Service Regions
1 Northern RHA, 2 Yorkshire RHA, 3 Trent RHA, 4 East Anglian RHA,
5 North West Thames RHA, 6 North East Thames RHA, 7 South East Thames
RHA, 8 South West Thames RHA, 9 Wessex RHA, 10 Oxford RHA, 11 South
Western RHA, 12 West Midlands RHA, 13 Mersey RHA, 14 North Western
RHA, 15 Wales

usually carried out by DHAs subject to the approval and guidance of
the RHA.
8　The blood transfusion service.

The chairman and members of each RHA are appointed by the Secretary of State after consultation with the universities, the larger local authorities and the main health professions. Members serve for four years with one half retiring every two years. The chairman receives payment on a part-time basis. Members are not paid but are entitled to travelling and other expenses. There are usually doctors and nurses on an RHA, but there will always be a majority of non-medical members. No current member of any District Team of Officers within that RHA can be a member of that RHA.

Officers of the Regional Health Authority (RHA)

There are five senior officers who form the Regional Team of Officers (RTO):

> Regional Medical Officer
> Regional Nursing Officer
> Regional Works Officer
> Regional Administrator
> Regional Treasurer

Each member of the RTO is of equal standing; one acts as chairman on a rotating basis. Although the RTO monitors the performance of the various District Teams of Officers within the Region, it is *not* managerially in charge of them.

The RTO is responsible for recommending regional policies to the RHA. This is done by the preparation of a *Regional Development Plan* which deals with:

(a) the distribution of medical specialities;
(b) development of medical and nursing manpower;
(c) the scheduling of major capital developments.

In addition, the RTO is very much concerned with monitoring the programmes of its DHAs and carefully reviews DHA planning and budget proposals.

District Health Authorities (DHAs)

There are 192 District Health Authorities (DHAs) in England.

Generally DHAs are responsible for the main day to day management of the local health services except the general practitioners.

The DHA is responsible for all the hospital and community health services and is in charge of:

District General Hospitals and other hospitals
Maternity and child health services
Domiciliary midwifery
Health visiting
Home nursing
Vaccination and immunization
Prevention of disease, care and after care (health education, chiropody, tuberculosis after care, occupational therapy and some types of convalescence)
School health services (in conjunction with the corresponding local education authority)

Nineteen of the DHAs also act as centres for medical teaching (in conjunction with the medical schools of the corresponding university). This extra responsibility is reflected in higher rates of remuneration to the members of the DTO. In addition all DHAs which act as centres for medical teaching are responsible for all consultants and senior registrar appointments. (In the rest of the health service such appointments are undertaken by the RHA.)

The chairman of each DHA is appointed by the Secretary of State while the members are appointed from the corresponding local authorities, university and by the RHA after consultation with the main health professions and other organizations. There is always a minority of doctors and nurses on any DHA.

District Team of Officers (DTO)

Each District Health Authority is serviced by a District Team of Officers (DTO) which consists of:

District Medical Officer
District Nursing Officer
District Administrator
District Treasurer
Two clinicians (one consultant and one general practitioner)

The DTO acts as the planning and evaluation team of the DHA. The team draws up planning guidelines and reviews and monitors performances within the district. It also advises the DHA on the development of health services in the district. The members of the DTO are of equal standing and each acts as chairman in rotation.

The main function of the DTO is to manage and co-ordinate all the main local hospital and community health services. Each District will have working within it all types of clinicians in consultant practice, as well as a unified hospital and community nursing service covering all aspects— general nursing, midwifery in hospitals and the community, psychiatric nursing, health visiting and home nursing services. There are also *various specialists in community medicine* working in the district although each DHA has the responsibility of deciding how these functions will be distributed between the local specialists in community medicine.

The DTO has to draw up and administer a budget for the DHA following advice from the District Treasurer.

Specialists in community medicine and community nursing

Although each DHA has to decide the allocation of duties between its specialists in community medicine, the following tasks have to be undertaken:

1 The giving of medical and nursing advice to the relevant local education authority on child health and school health matters. It is expected that most DHAs will appoint staff equivalent to the former Specialists in Community (Child Health) and Area Nurse (Child Health) to assist in the organization and management of the school health service.

2 The giving of medical advice to the relevant local authority on environmental health matters. Such a doctor will also have to act as '*proper officer*' to each local authority in the District who has environmental health responsibilities. Such a Specialist in Community Medicine also helps to control outbreaks of communicable diseases or food poisoning and works closely with the environmental health officers of the local authorities. Notification of communicable and infectious diseases are reported by the patient's doctor to the 'proper officer'. In the cases of outbreaks of infectious diseases the 'proper officer' has, for the purpose of carrying out an epidemiological investigation, executive control over environmental health officers, port health inspectors or health visitors as regards that investigation.

Health-Care Planning Teams

Health-Care Planning Teams are multi-disciplinary working parties of officers set up in each District to analyse and assess the needs of the health services. There are two types of Health-Care Planning Teams:

1   permanent teams continuously dealing with the following:
       children
       maternity services
       mentally ill
       mentally handicapped
       elderly

2 'ad hoc' teams set up specially to consider a special subject. Such teams may be disbanded after they have studied and reported on a specific subject. They cover many aspects and examples include:
   review of primary health care services
   introduction of day surgery in hospitals
   diagnosis, treatment and prevention of non-accidental injury in babies.

Each Health-Care Planning Team contains a wide range of professionals in the health service—general practitioners, consultants, hospital and community nursing staff (midwives, home nurses and health visitors), para-medical staff—radiographers, physiotherapists, occupational therapists, chiropodists, hospital social workers from the corresponding local authority. The Health-Care Planning Teams provide an opportunity for views on special subjects within each district to be studied in detail and to be presented to the District Team of Officers and from there to the District Health Authority and Regional Health Authority and to the Department of Health and Social Security. The District Health Authority through the Joint Consultative Committee (see below) will discuss with the local authority the views of the Health-Care Planning Teams.

Joint Care Planning—Health and Local Authorities

Because services provided by local authorities (particularly those of the social services departments) have a considerable impact on health services and vice versa, it has been decided by the Department of Health and Social Security that effective arrangements should be made for joint planning.
   Joint Care Planning Teams have therefore been set up by all District Health Authorities and the relevant local authorities (including social services and education departments). Joint planning will cover all aspects of health and social services but is particularly important to ensure the correct balance of services for the elderly, the disabled, the mentally handicapped, the mentally ill, children and families and for socially handicapped groups such as alcoholics and drug addicts.

Joint Consultative Committees

Every District Health Authority and the matching local authority/authorities must set up a *Joint Consultative Committee* (JCC) which has the responsibility of advising on the planning and operation of the health services and the social, environmental and education services run by the local authority. The aim of such a committee is to improve co-operation.

Community Health Councils

Community Health Councils were introduced into the health service by the National Health Service (Reorganization) Act, 1973. There is approximately one for each District. Their main function is to represent the local consumers' interests and to ensure that the development of the local health service does take regard of local opinion. Each contains 18–30 members, one third of whom are drawn from voluntary bodies active within the district. About half the members are appointed by the corresponding local authority and one sixth by the Regional Health Authority (who provide any permanent staff). No member of a Regional Health Authority, District Health Authority, Family Practitioner Committee, nor any doctor or other National Health Service employee may serve on a Community Health Council.

Each Community Health Council has the following list of matters which it can investigate:

1 the effectiveness of the health services in that District
2 planning of health services
3 variations in local health services—closure of hospitals or hospital departments
4 collaboration between the health services and the local authority environmental health, education and social services
5 standards of service—number of hospital beds in the district and the average number of patients on family doctors' lists
6 patient facilities including hospital out-patients, open visiting of children, waiting times, amenities for hospital patients and arrangements for rehabilitation of patients
7 waiting periods for in-patients' and out-patients' treatments and for domiciliary services
8 quality of catering in hospitals and in other health service institutions
9 complaints (*not* individual complaints from patients, see below, but the general type of complaint)
10 advice to individual members of the public on how and where they should lodge a complaint and the facts that should be provided.

Each Community Health Council must issue an annual report which must then be sent to the Regional Health Authority and District Health Authority. It is hoped that these Community Health Councils will provide a chance for local people using the health services to keep a careful watch over their development.

General Practitioner services

Family Practitioner Committee

A special committee called the Family Practitioner Committee is responsible to the Department of Health and Social Security on all matters concerning the local family doctor services, the dental services and the optical and pharmaceutical services. All these professionals are independent contractors and hold their contracts with the Family Practitioner Committee.

In November 1981, the Government announced that legislation would be introduced to separate completely these services from the DHAs so that in future, the Family Practitioner Committee will be completely responsible for such services.

Each Family Practitioner Committee contains 30 members, half of whom are appointed by the professions and the remainder by the local health authorities and local authorities.

There is a special machinery set up nationally by the Secretary of State—the *Medical Practices Committee*—which is constantly assessing the number of general practitioners in any area compared with its population. It then classifies each area into one of four types:

(i) *Designated area*—an area in which there is an inadequate number of doctors, where the average number of patients per doctor exceeds 2500. Doctors are encouraged to practise in such an area and will receive a special inducement payment.

(ii) *Open area*—an area with a fair number of doctors where the doctor/patient ratio is between 1/2100 and 1/2500. Permission will always be granted to practise in such an area.

(iii) *Intermediate area*—an area with the doctor/patient ratio between 1/1800 and 1/2100. Applications to practise in such areas will never automatically be granted and each area is considered on its merits with special reference to the trends in the area.

(iv) *Restricted area*—an area which is over-doctored and where the number of patients per doctor is below 1/1800. Permission is never granted to start a new practice in a Restricted Area and entry can only be obtained by applying for a vacancy or partnership or assistantship.

Size of practice and choice of patient and doctor

A limit of 3500 is fixed on the total number of patients any single doctor may have on his list. If the doctor employs an assistant (he must have the permission of the Family Practitioner Committee to do this), the limit is raised by a further 2000 patients.

The public have a completely free choice of doctor and the doctor also has a free choice of deciding whether or not to accept a patient on to his list. Once the patient has been accepted by the doctor, he is required to render to him all proper and necessary treatment. If the doctor has also agreed to give maternity medical services, then this treatment will include such services for which he will receive additional payment. In addition the doctor must arrange further medical treatment for his patients such as the admission to hospital or attendance at out-patients. Every general practitioner is responsible for ensuring adequate medical cover during his absence on holiday or for sickness.

Medical List

Each Family Practitioner Committee is required to keep a list of all doctors practising in the area, called the *Medical List*, which must indicate separately the general medical practitioners who undertake maternity services. This list is available at the local Family Practitioner Committee headquarters and main Post Offices, where it may be examined by any member of the public to help in his choice of a doctor.

If a patient has difficulty in finding a doctor to accept him, he can apply to the Allocation Committee (another sub-committee of the Family Practitioner Committee) which will then allocate the patient to a convenient doctor. There are facilities for a patient to change his doctor if he wishes to do so, or for a doctor to indicate that he no longer wishes to look after a particular patient.

Methods of controlling local general medical practice

Local Medical Committee. One of the most important committees of any Family Practitioner Committee is the *Local Medical Committee* of doctors which acts as the local medical advisory committee to the Family Practitioner Committee. Any difficulties connected with particular practices or with local policies are referred to the Local Medical Committee who then advises the Family Practitioner Committee. In the case of a doctor who is considered by the Secretary of State to be prescribing excessive drugs and appliances for his patients, the Local Medical Committee has the task of carrying out an investigation. If, as a result of their enquiry, the Local Medical Committee come to the conclusion that there has been excessive prescribing, then they must report the case to the Family Practitioner Committee who may then recommend the Secretary of State for Social Services to withhold a certain sum from the remuneration of the doctor, as a penalty. Usually such action is rarely taken, a warning first being given to the doctor.

Other similar expert committees help in the administration of the dental service—the *Dental Service Committee*, with the pharmaceutical services—the *Area Chemists Contractors Committee*, or with the ophthalmic services—the *Ophthalmic Service Committee*.

Methods of controlling general practice

A *Medical Services Committee* appointed by the Family Practitioner Committee investigates any serious complaints raised by a patient about the services to him by his doctor. This consists of the Chairman of the Family Practitioner Committee plus six other members of which three must be from the Local Medical Committee. There is a set procedure laid down for the investigation of such complaints. Minor complaints can be investigated by the Administrator to the Family Practitioner Committee and major complaints by the Medical Services Committee. Also the hearing is always in private and the doctor's name is never made public. The Medical Services Committee reports its findings to the Family Practitioner Committee which then sends its decision to the Secretary of State. The doctor may also appeal to the Secretary of State. In the case of a proved complaint, a doctor may be warned, have a special limit as to the number of patients on his list imposed, or have a sum withheld from his remuneration. There is no appeal beyond the Secretary of State whose decision is final.

In very serious cases, the Family Practitioner Committee can refer the case to a central *Tribunal* set up by the Secretary of State for Social Services, with a chairman who must be a barrister or solicitor of at least ten years' standing. The Tribunal holds an inquiry and, if satisfied that the case is serious enough, can order the removal of the doctor *from general practice in the Health Service*. In such a case, there is a right of appeal to the Secretary of State. This is quite different from action by the General Medical Council which can determine the fitness for a doctor to practice in *any medical field*.

Value of general medical services

There is little doubt that, although the hospital and specialist services cost so much more, the standard of medical service provided for each individual patient depends as much on the standard of the general medical services as on any other factor. Although there is no compulsion on any person to register with a doctor, the vast majority of people have so registered—about 98–99 per cent of the population.

Charges to patients

There is no additional cost to the individual in obtaining all the medical services provided by hospitals or by general practitioners. Some charges are levied for prescription. Prescriptions for the following people can be obtained without charge by completing the declaration on the back of the prescription form: children aged 16 years and under, women aged 60 and over and men aged 65 and over, and people holding exemption certificates. These are issued to expectant and nursing mothers, people suffering from certain medical conditions, persons and their dependents receiving supplementary benefit and family income supplement. A part charge is made for all dental treatment and other charges are levied for dentures, but these are free for young persons (anyone under 16 or in full-time attendance at school) and expectant and nursing mothers. Charges are also made for spectacles.

Health Service Commissioners

Health Service Commissioners for England and Wales were introduced by the National Health Service Reorganization Act, 1973, to investigate complaints against the relevant health bodies.

Both these commissioners are only removable on an address from both Houses of Parliament and their salaries are paid directly out of the Consolidated Fund. They are therefore in the same independent position as High Court Judges.

The main functions of these Health Service Commissioners are to investigate:

1 An alleged failure in a service provided by a relevant health body— Regional Health Authority, District Health Authority, Family Practitioner Committee, Public Health Laboratory Service Board or any special body appointed before and after 1 April 1974.
2 An alleged failure of a relevant body to provide a service which it was a function of that body to provide.
3 Any other act taken by or on behalf of a relevant body in a case where it is alleged any person has sustained injustice or hardship in consequence of the failure or of maladministration.

It is important to note that the Health Service Commissioner is specifically excluded from dealing with:

1 Professional complaints against decisions of individual doctors or nurses in regard to individual patients.
2 Any action which is dealt with by the tribunal set up to deal with serious complaints (see page 15).
3 Any complaint which is subject to action in a court of law.

Scotland

The Scottish Home and Health Department is responsible to the Secretary of State for Scotland for the administration of the National

Health Service in Scotland. Its head office is at New St Andrews House, Edinburgh.

There are 15 local health boards in Scotland which administer on behalf of the Secretary of State for health services in Scotland (other than those carried out by the Common Services Agency—see below). These boards take the major policy decisions such as the allocation of resources and the long term planning of services. However, many day to day decisions are taken by the chief officers of each health board working together as an executive group.

The Secretary of State for Scotland is responsible to Parliament and there is a Scottish Health Service Planning Council set up to advise the Secretary of State on:

(a) the identification of health priorities in relation to the resources available and the necessary measures to meet them;

(b) the implementation, review and evaluation of health planning in Scotland's national health services;

(c) the integration of health care with other kinds of care to ensure a coordinated policy for the treatment of people in need.

To assist it, the Council has set up a number of Advisory Groups.

An interesting difference in Scotland is that a central body—the Common Services Agency—has been set up to provide on behalf of the Secretary of State and the health boards a range of specialized services which are more effectively organized on a national basis including dental estimates, ambulance and blood transfusion services, the buying of equipment and other supplies, the planning and design of health service buildings, legal services and health education. Responsibility for the administration of these services rests with a management committee appointed by the Secretary of State. The Common Services Agency whose headquarters are at Trinity Park House, Edinburgh, has a number of separate units including the Scottish Health Services Council, the Scottish Health Education Unit, the Communicable Diseases (Scotland) Unit, the central Legal Office of the health services in Scotland and the Information Services Division.

In addition there are:

1 a series of *local area consultative committees* to advise health boards on the provision of services in their area. These represent doctors, dentists, pharmacists and ophthalmic and dispensing opticians and advise on all professional matters.

2 *university liaison committees* which advise on undergraduate and postgraduate teaching and on research.

3 a series of 48 *local health councils* which represent the 'consumer' interests of patients.

In the Scottish Health services much emphasis has been laid on *integration of services for patients* and not only at senior management level. Services are planned mainly to meet the needs of patients and to make the best possible use of the staff, money and physical resources. Team work in all aspects of the health services is stressed as well as the involvement of doctors and clinical workers in management matters.

Wales

There are important differences between the health services in England and Wales for no regional tier of health authorities has been set up in Wales.

The Secretary of State for Wales has overall authority to Parliament for the health services in Wales and has four main duties:

1 to determine the health policies in Wales
2 to allocate resources between the nine District Health Authorities in Wales
3 to ensure that the objectives of the services are achieved
4 to ensure that the standards of the health services in Wales are satisfactory.

There are nine District Health Authorities in Wales: (a) Dyfed, (b) Clwyd, (c) Gwent, (d) Gwynedd, (e) Mid Glamorgan, (f) Powys, (g) South Glamorgan, (h) West Glamorgan, (i) West Dyfed. These DHAs are responsible to the Secretary of State for Wales for all the day to day health services (with the exception of those carried out by the Welsh Health Technical Services Organization—see below). District Teams of Officers (DTOs) function in very similar ways to those in England with the addition that a senior member of each health profession is appointed locally to give advice to the DTO and to the DHA about all matters which are relevant to his/her profession.

The *Welsh Health Technical Services Organization* is directly accountable to the Secretary of State for Wales and has three main functions:

1 the designing and building of all major hospital and other capital works for the health services in Wales
2 the control and running of a central computer service for the health services in Wales
3 the negotiation of all central supply contracts for health services in Wales.

2
The Measurement of Health

The measurement or assessment of the health of a community is an important feature of any preventive health programme. Rarely is it possible to attempt to carry out all desirable preventive health work in any area at once. It is, therefore, essential to be able to assess the fluctuations in the health of the community from time to time, and to decide which are the worst problems so that they may be tackled first. It is also valuable to be able to compare the health of say one city or country with another. Often, in this way, marked variations will be shown in the health of different places and then a search can be started to discover the reasons behind such differences.

The assessment of the health of any group of individuals may occasionally be made by a series of medical examinations held on all the people in say a factory or a school. But this is only possible where there is complete control over the persons involved and is never practicable for a whole community such as a city, town or country. The measurement of the health of such populations is only possible by indirect methods, by studying various factors such as mortality of the population from different diseases and studies of the incidence of disease. The collection and interpretation of such information is called the study of *Vital Statistics*.

Most of these studies concern either the incidence of disease (*morbidity*) or the proportion of persons within the community dying from disease (*mortality*). Although accurate records of incidence of disease are the more valuable, it is rarely possible to get such figures as there is no method of ensuring that all or even a fixed proportion of cases are reported. It is, however, necessary to know the cause of all deaths (for legal purposes), and mortality statistics are usually very complete and certainly more reliable when dealing with very large communities. But even with mortality statistics, difficulties may arise from different standards of diagnosis and from the introduction of a new form of treatment which may change the mortality completely. An example of this is typhoid fever. The mortality rate of this disease has fallen over 10 per cent to less than 1 per cent following the introduction of ampicillin treatment. Thus, the present mortality rate cannot be used as a reliable indicator of the incidence of this disease.

It is obviously desirable to refer to all statistics in terms of the same unit of population and this is normally per 1000 or per 100 000 persons. Thus the *Crude Death Rate* is the number of persons who *die per year per 1000 persons*. The *Infant Mortality Rate* is the number of infants under the age of 1 year who die per 1000 births per year. The *Maternal Mortality Rate* is the number of women who die from causes associated with childbirth *per 100 000 total births.*

It is essential to know the population accurately to calculate these various death rates. A *Census*—when the population is counted—is undertaken every ten years and was last carried out in April 1981. The Registrar General calculates the estimated population of all areas in the intermediate years between each Census.

Age distribution of the population

The distribution of the various age groups within the population is of interest:

Table 2.1   Age and structure of Population, England and Wales 1983 (mid-year)

	Males		*Females*		*Total*	
Age Group	Thousands	Per cent	Thousands	Per cent	Thousands	Per cent
·0–14	5091.6	21.0	4730.3	18.5	9721.9	19.5
15–44	10 784.6	44.5	10 546.2	41.4	21 330.8	43.0
45–64	5451.0	22.5	5649.6	22.2	11 100.6	22.5
65–74	1932.8	7.9	2483.0	9.7	4415.8	8.9
75–84	883.4	0.5	439.6	1.7	572.3	1.1

(from O.P.C.S Monitor PP1 84/3)

Note that although there are larger numbers of males in the population at the younger age groups, the reverse occurs in old age—there are many more old women alive than old men. In 1983 there were 133 700 men aged 85 years and over compared with more than three times as many women—439 600.

The proportion of old people in the population has been rising steadily throughout this century. In 1901 only 4.7 per cent of the community was aged 65 years and over compared with 15 per cent today.

The **Birth Rate** is the number of children born per year 1000 of the population. This is affected by many factors such as the numbers of persons of reproductive age within a population—the higher their proportion, the higher is likely to be the birth rate. The social habits of a country will cause great changes in birth rate—the rate in Poland (a predominantly Roman Catholic country) is 19.5 (1979) compared with a rate in England and Wales for the same year of 11.6. A rapidly developing country will usually show a high birth rate—e.g. Israel whose rate in 1979 was 24.7.

The accompanying graph of the Birth Rate in England and Wales from 1900 to present day (Fig. 2.1) shows many fascinating changes. It will be

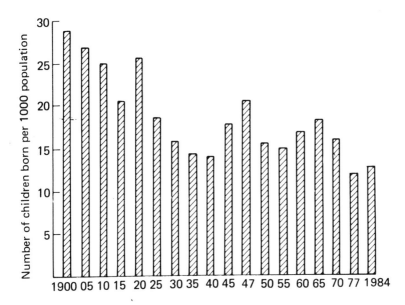

Fig. 2.1   Birth rate, England and Wales

seen that the rate fell steadily to the very low figure of 14.4 in 1933; it fell during the Second World War, rose to a peak in 1947, and fell again, only to rise once more to the figure of 18.5 in 1964. Since that year, it fell steadily to 11.6 in 1977, increased again to 13.0 in 1979, but then fell to 12.8 in 1984.

These changes tell one much about the pattern of human life in those 84 years. The high rate in 1900 was associated with a very high death rate among children (15 per cent died before their first birthday) so that although the birth rate was high a much smaller proportion of children reached adult life than today. The low rate of the 1930s was connected with the very unstable living conditions between the two world wars. The 1947 peak was the result of many families being re-united after the war. The 1965 high figure is dependent upon many factors, including earlier marriage and greater prosperity. During the last fifteen years, increasing use of effective contraceptives (the pill), abortion and less prosperity have all played an important part in reducing the birth rate.

The most recent rise is due mainly to technical reasons, there being a higher proportion of persons of child bearing age in the community caused by the high birth rates in the 1947–55 period.

The **Crude Death Rate** (the number of persons dying per 1000 population) is of little value, as the relative population in towns is never known accurately. When there is a large number of aged inhabitants, the number of deaths in such a community is bound to be higher, irrespective of the living conditions in that area. More important is the **Standardized**

Community Health and Social Services

Table 2.2 Deaths by selected causes. Standardized Mortality Ratios, England, 1980 (1968 = 100)

Cause	Sex	SMR
All causes	Male	87
	Female	88
Tuberculosis (respiratory)	Male	34
Hyperplasia of the prostate	Male	37
Hypertensive diseases	Female	41
Tuberculosis (respiratory)	Female	47
Bronchitis	Male	48
Meningeal infections	Male	52
Cancer of stomach	Female	72
Cancer of cervix uteri	Female	82
Suicide	Female	86
Ischaemic heart disease	Male	98
Cancer of the breast	Female	112
Ulcer of the stomach	Female	146
Cancer of the lung	Female	159
Nephritis and nephrosis	Female	195

(from Health and Personal Social Service Statistics, DHSS, 1982)

Mortality Ratio (SMR) which makes allowances for changes in the age structure of the population (1968 = 100). In 1980 the SMR was 87.

Table 2.2 gives the SMRs for selected diseases for England for 1980.

It will be seen that from 1968 to 1980 many unequal changes occurred in mortality. Deaths from childbirth and abortion have fallen by almost two thirds, hyperplasia of prostate, hypertensive diseases and bronchitis by almost one third, ischaemic heart disease and cancer of lung in males have increased very slightly, but death from cancer of the lung in women has increased by over one half.

The **Infant Mortality Rate** is one of the most useful death rates to give an indication of the living conditions of any area. The infant mortality rate is the number of infants who die under 1 year of age per 1000 live related births. It is a measure of the number of children who die before reaching their first birthday per 1000 born alive. In 1983 in England and Wales the rate was 10.0 which means that 1.00 per cent of infants born alive, died in their first year of life.

The improvement in the infant mortality rate, and consequently in the living conditions in England and Wales, is shown in Table 2.3.

If a graph is drawn of this improvement (see Fig. 2.2), it will be seen that there has been a general improvement throughout the last eighty years. There have, however, been periods such as the 1930s when the change was very slow due to the slowing down of the improvement in the living conditions. The infant mortality rate is a sensitive indicator of changes in the living conditions. It can, for instance, be used to compare the living

Table 2.3 Infant Mortality Rate per 1000 live births, (England and Wales) 1900–1983

1900	138
1910	112
1920	84
1930	60
1940	56
1950	29.6
1960	21.8
1965	19.0
1970	18.2
1974	16.3
1975	15.7
1979	12.8
1983	10.0

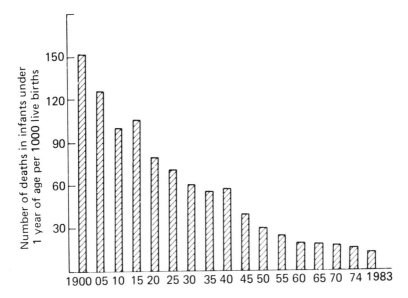

Fig. 2.2 Infant Mortality Rate, England and Wales, 1900–1983

conditions of large cities in the same country. The rates for many large towns in England were as shown in Table 2.4.

Many people find it difficult to believe that the excellent paediatric services available in some cities do not improve matters. They do play their part in keeping the deaths lower than they might otherwise be, but the main factors affecting an infant's health are the conditions in the home. An increase of unemployment leading to deterioration of living conditions would increase infant deaths. Indeed a political decision which

Table 2.4   Infant Mortality Rate per 1000 live births, 1979

Bromley	9.7
Stockport	9.7
Reading	9.8
Redbridge (London)	10.7
Liverpool	11.4
Bristol	13.5
Wakefield	16.1
Manchester	18.5
Calderdale	21.2

Table 2.5   Infant mortality rates in different countries, 1977

Sweden	8.0	USA	14.0
Denmark	8.7	Germany	
Japan	8.9	(Federal)	15.5
Netherlands	9.5	Israel	17.8
France	11.5	USSR	27.7
Canada	12.4	Romania	31.2
England & Wales	13.8	Yugoslavia	35.2
		Portugal	38.9

reduced unemployment might do more to prevent infant deaths than many medical improvements.

There are wide variations between the infant mortality rates of different countries of the world (Table 2.5).

An important part of the infant mortality rate is the number of infant deaths which occur in the first four weeks of life—the **Neonatal Mortality Rate**. In 1983 this was 5.8 per 1000 live related births showing that two thirds of the first year deaths occur within the first 4 weeks of life.

The majority of neonatal deaths occur in the first week of life and this is now called the early neonatal mortality rate. Thus in 1983 the neonatal mortality rate was made up as follows:

Early neonatal mortality rate	4.7
Late neonatal mortality rate	1.1
	5.8

The **Perinatal Mortality Rate** is a combination of the number of *stillbirths* and of *deaths* that occur within the first week of life, per 1000 total births—early neonatal death rate.

In 1983, in England and Wales, the perinatal mortality rate was 10.4 (5.7 stillbirth rate plus 4.7 deaths in the first week of life).

Table 2.6 Perinatal Mortality, England and Wales, 1950–83

1950	37.4
1955	37.4
1960	32.8
1965	26.9
1970	23.5
1971	22.3
1974	20.5
1975	19.0
1979	14.7
1983	10.4

The value of the perinatal mortality rate is that it gives a very good indication of the hazards to a baby immediately before and after birth. The gradual fall of the perinatal mortality is shown in Table 2.6.

The **Maternal Mortality Rate** is another very interesting death rate which is the number of women who die from causes associated with childbirth per 100 000 total births. It is a measure of the risk attached to childbirth, as deaths are only counted if they are directly related to the pregnancy.

Examination of the maternal mortality rate shows that since 1900 it has improved dramatically. In 1979 it was 12 compared with 481 in 1900.

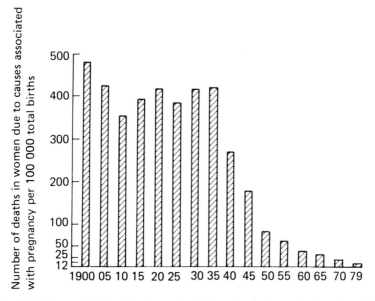

Fig. 2.3 Maternal Mortality Rate (including abortion), England and Wales, 1900–79

But examination of the way in which this rate has improved shows that it did so quite differently compared with the infant mortality rate. Comparison of the two graphs shows that the infant mortality rate gradually and steadily improved throughout the last eighty years, whereas the maternal mortality rate hardly altered from 1900 to 1930 and at the beginning of the 1930s had actually risen to 410. It then fell very quickly after 1937. The reason for this difference is that the maternal mortality rate is affected by entirely different factors—whereas the infant mortality rate is mainly connected with living conditions, *the maternal mortality rate is related to the standard of obstetric practice.* An advance in obstetrics, particularly the introduction of chemotherapy and antibiotics, cut down the dangers of deaths from puerperal infection dramatically after 1937. It was later followed by further advances reducing the danger of toxaemias and haemorrhage.

The way in which these statistics have helped to suggest improvements in obstetrics and thus prevent much illness is described in detail in the next chapter.

Studies into the incidence of disease

Morbidity measurement

Many different methods of measuring the incidence of disease (morbidity) are currently being perfected. Some of the most interesting of these have been connected with hospital records in special studies now undertaken called Hospital In-Patient Enquiry and Hospital Activity Analysis. Studies have also concentrated upon the certificates of sickness received from general practitioners. Examples of these are now given in Table 2.7.

There are broad similarities in the discharge pattern of both sexes. The number of women exceed men but this excess is greater in mental illness (37%) than in physical illness (13%). Digestive system, respiratory and heart disease are all greater in men, but disease of the breast and female genital system are the largest cause in women and represent at 1020 admissions a much larger figure than male genital disorders (335). Note also that 'other neoplasms' and 'endocrine, nutritional and metabolic disease' figure among the 15 commonest causes in women but not in men.

Another interesting method of illustrating statistics is given in the diagram (Fig. 2.4, p. 28) demonstrating the average number of beds occupied daily in hospitals in Great Britain in 1977.

This diagram emphasizes the large number of hospital beds occupied by mental disability, 42.4 per cent (mental illness 27.2 per cent and mental impairment 15.2 per cent). Although in number of discharges (see Table 2.7) pregnancy is the largest in women, the total maternity beds

Table 2.7 Diagnostic statistics in non-psychiatric hospitals, England, 1978

Cause	No.
Males	
1 Symptoms and ill defined conditions	1126
2 Diseases of the digestive system	1000
3 Diseases of the respiratory system	887
4 Other injuries and reactions	831
5 Rheumatic fever, hypertensive disease and heart disease	662
6 Cancer	659
7 Diseases of the peripheral circulatory system	472
8 Fractures, dislocations and sprains	432
9 Diseases of the musculoskeletal system	357
10 Male genital disorders	325
11 Diseases of the eye	191
12 Infective and parasitic diseases (including tuberculosis)	179
13 Congenital anomalies	179
14 Diseases of the skin	156
15 Diseases of the urinary system	153
Females	
1 Symptoms and ill defined conditions	1166
2 Diseases of the breast and female genital system	890
3 Diseases of the digestive system	835
4 Diseases of the respiratory system	653
5 Cancer	622
6 Other injuries and reactions	612
7 Diseases of the peripheral circulatory system	472
8 Rheumatic fever, hypertensive disease and heart disease	459
9 Diseases of the musculoskeletal system	426
10 Fractures, dislocations and sprains	364
11 Benign neoplasms	316
12 Endocrine, nutritional and metabolic diseases	219
13 Diseases of the eye	213
14 Diseases of the nervous system	199
15 Infective and parasitic diseases (including tuberculosis)	148

(from Health and Personal Social Service Statistics DHSS, 1982)

number only 4 per cent due to the short stay in hospital of many such cases.

An analysis of the causes of sickness certified is another useful way of studying disease morbidity. The following tables are taken from the Digest of Health Statistics for England and Wales published by the Department of Health and Social Security.

There are two main ways of presenting such returns:

1 new spells of sickness (rate per 1000 at risk (Table 2.8, p. 29))
2 days of sickness per 1000 persons at risk (Table 2.9, p. 30)

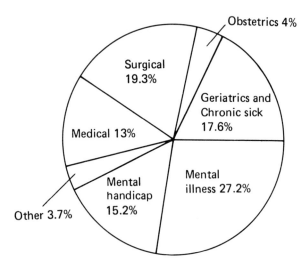

Fig. 2.4 Average number of beds occupied daily by cause, Great Britain, 1977

It is most interesting to compare these tables both for differences between the sexes and to see how, in some diseases, although the number of spells of sickness is smaller, the days lost are very large. Ischaemic heart disease is not among the 12 commonest causes of new spells of sickness, but is third in importance in days lost in males and ninth in females. The importance of mental illness in women is once more emphasized, being first in days lost in women (fourth in men) and seventh in spells of sickness in women (eleventh in men). Bronchitis causes more than twice the number of days lost in men (1844) compared with women (811). Diseases of the digestive system, influenza, and unspecified (symptoms and ill-defined) are very similar in both sexes. Disease of the urinary system and of the breast and genital systems do not appear in either sex (are fourteenth in women).

Communicable diseases

Before any effective preventive measures can be planned, it is essential to know the levels of incidence of the disease in question.

Most serious communicable diseases must be notified to the 'proper officer'. This will normally be the appropriate Community Physician or District Medical Officer. This allows the disease to be completely investigated and its source of infection discovered, as well as allowing a complete record of the incidence of the disease to be maintained.

Table 2.8 The 12 commonest causes of new spells of certified incapacity (rate per 1000 persons at risk, Great Britain, 1975)

	Cause	*No.*
Males		
1.	Other diseases of respiratory system	79.4
2.	Influenza	47.8
3.	Symptoms and ill-defined	44.9
4.	Infections and parasitic diseases	38.5
5.	Accidents	34.1
6.	Disease of digestive system ⎫	33.7
7.	Bronchitis ⎭	
8.	Sprains and strains (joints)	23.5
9.	Arthritis	23.3
10.	Other diseases of musculoskeletal system	19.1
11.	Mental illness	13.9
12.	Skin diseases	11.5

	Cause	*No.*
Females		
1.	Other diseases of respiratory system	125.1
2.	Symptoms and ill-defined	70.5
3.	Influenza	49.9
4.	Infections and parasitic diseases	48.8
5.	Complications of pregnancy	26.8
6.	Diseases of digestive system	25.8
7.	Bronchitis ⎫	25.4
	Mental illness ⎭	
9.	Accidents	21.8
10.	Diseases of urinary system	15.0
11.	Arthritis	14.7
12.	Other diseases of musculoskeletal system	12.9

(from *Health and Personal Social Services Statistics*, DHSS, 1977)

Table 2.9   The 12 commonest causes of working days lost (rate per 1000 persons at risk), Great Britain, 1975

Cause	*Days lost*
Males	
1. Bronchitis	1844
2. Symptoms and ill-defined	1745
3. Ischaemic heart disease	1728
4. Mental illness	1374
5. Other diseases of respiratory system	1185
6. Arthritis	1167
7. Other diseases of circulatory system	1052
8. Diseases of digestive system	1026
9. Accidents	896
10. Diseases of nervous system	859
11. Other diseases of musculoskeletal system	713
12. Influenza	494
Females	
1. Mental illness	2460
2. Symptoms and ill-defined	2234
3. Other diseases of respiratory system	1451
4. Arthritis	1276
5. Complications of pregnancy	1261
6. Diseases of nervous system	904
7. Bronchitis	811
8. Other diseases of circulatory system	798
9. Ischaemic heart disease	709
10. Diseases of digestive system	701
11. Infections and parasitic diseases	601
12. Other diseases of musculoskeletal system	532

(from *Health and Personal Social Services Statistics*, DHSS, 1977)

The statistics in Table 2.10 show that diphtheria is no longer a problem and also illustrates the success of the immunization scheme introduced in 1942 and continued ever since.

Another interesting record is the fall of new cases of *tuberculosis* over the last 31 years as shown in Table 2.11.

A useful feature which these records also emphasize is that the *problem of tuberculosis in men and women is changing in proportion*. In 1950, the ratio of male and female cases was 1.2 to 1. But by 1964, the cases in women had fallen much faster and now the ratio is 2.0 to 1.0, men to women. By 1981, it had changed again to 1.6 to 1.0. An accurate knowledge of how the problem changes is essential to ensure that

Table 2.10 Diphtheria, England and Wales, 1942–83

Year	No. of cases notified	
1942	41 404	←—Mass immunization
1943	34 662	programme started
1944	23 199	
1945	18 596	
1946	11 986	
1947	5 609	
1948	3 575	
1949	1 881	
1950	622	
1954	173	
1958	80	
1962	16	
1966	20	
1970	22	
1972	5	
1974	3	
1978	3	
1979	0	
1983	4	

Table 2.11 Notification of Pulmonary Tuberculosis, England and Wales, 1950–83

Year	Males	Females	Total
1950	26 969	22 389	49 358
1952	26 558	21 536	48 093
1954	23 694	18 654	42 348
1956	20 683	14 821	35 504
1958	17 955	11 883	29 838
1960	14 351	9 254	23 605
1962	11 749	6 096	17 845
1964	10 013	5 006	15 019
1966	8 257	4 109	12 366
1968	7 705	4 623	12 328
1970	6 998	4 282	11 280
1975	6 541	4 277	10 818
1983	3 291	2 026	5 317

preventive health measures are concentrated where they will be most useful. In the example given above, it is clear that more effort is now called for to attack the problem of tuberculosis in men than women.

Non-communicable disease

The value of a study into the incidence of non-communicable diseases is that it emphasizes the relative problems of different diseases and stimulates research into factors which are connected with their incidence. Very often special research studies are started in this way and lead to important preventive factors being demonstrated. A good example of this is given by *cancer of the lung*, which has increased so alarmingly from 6439 deaths in 1940 to 35 168 in 1980 (see Fig. 2.5) that research has been undertaken to find out the reasons for this increase. The Royal College of Physicians has studied this problem and their reports stated that cigarette smoking is an important cause of lung cancer. The latest report goes much further and indicates clearly the risks involved in cigarette smoking.

A recent report by the Independent Scientific Committee on Smoking and Health was published in 1979 and describes the work undertaken in relation to the inclusion of substitutes and additives in tobacco products, including the development of 'lower risk' cigarettes. The Committee believes that whereas no cigarette can ever be regarded as completely safe, cigarettes can be developed which give less concern than many current

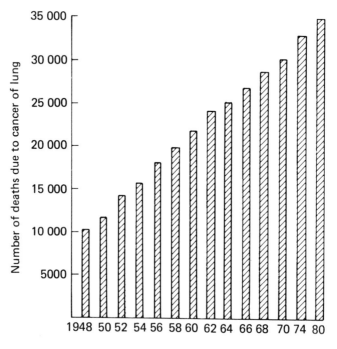

Fig. 2.5 Deaths from cancer of lung, England and Wales, 1948–80

brands, because they carry a lower risk to the cardio-vascular system. The aim will be to develop, in co-operation with the tobacco industry, cigarettes with a low yield of tar and carbon monoxide.

Although a study of the statistics of cancer of the lung shows that it could be reduced by persuading people to stop or not to start smoking, the actual ways in which the nation can be persuaded are more complex. The Department or Health and Social Security estimates that four out of every ten deaths in men (including those from heart and chest diseases) could be prevented by the abandonment of cigarette smoking.

Further studies using statistics have shown that cancer of the lung has also increased in city dwellers compared with those living in the country due to the excessive atmospheric pollution in cities. The differences are not nearly as great as between cigarette smokers and non-smokers but sufficient to lead to further research.

The incidence of *Ischaemic Heart Disease* is another problem in which statistics are being utilized widely in promoting research into possible causative factors. During the last twenty one years there has been a marked rise in the number of persons in England and Wales who die from this cause. The rise in the number of persons dying from ischaemic heart disease is startling as seen by the following table:

Table 2.12 Deaths from Ischaemic Heart Disease, England and Wales, 1961–83

Year	Males	Females	Total
1961	66 400	50 100	116 500
1966	75 300	54 800	130 100
1970	80 800	58 500	139 300
1983	89 524	67 026	156 550

It will be seen that recorded deaths from ischaemic heart disease have increased by nearly 50 per cent in the last 18 years. The actual increase may not be as great as suggested because:

1 the population in 1983 contains a larger proportion of elderly people and this group is one in which death from ischaemic heart disease is high;
2 the level of diagnosis may have improved.

To make certain that all factors are understood, investigations are taking place into the incidence of ischaemic heart disease. Many different factors are being investigated, such as the effect of increased exercise, diet or the stature of individuals. Many of these researches will take a long time to complete but it is hoped that they will eventually lead to a better understanding of the factors which cause ischaemic heart disease and to methods of preventing it.

Social factors in disease

A further method that can be employed to study disease is to compare the mortality of illness by grouping the family by occupation. The Registrar General divides the population in England and Wales into six different *social classes* based on the occupation of the chief wage earner of the family.

Non-Manual

Class I	Professional occupations (lawyers, doctors etc.).
Class II	Managerial and lower professional occupations (i.e. teachers, nurses, sales managers).
Class III N	Non-manual skilled occupations (clerks, shop assistants).

Manual

Class III M	Skilled manual occupations (bricklayers, underground coal miners etc.)
Class IV	Partly skilled occupations (bus conductors, postmen etc.)
Class V	Unskilled occupations (porters, labourers etc.).

The latest publication illustrating the mortality of different occupations was published in 1978 (Occupational Mortality 1970–72 OPCS). The results are given in the form called the *Standardised Mortality Ratio (SMR)*. This is given as a ratio 100. A group experiencing exactly the expected mortality would have an SMR of 100. If the SMR was 75, then the group has 75/100 or 3/4 of the expected mortality (it is enjoying less mortality than expected). If the SMR is 200, it means that the mortality is 200/100 or twice as great as normal.

Table 2.13 shows the wider variations in mortality between the different social classes.

It is interesting to note that generally social classes I and II enjoy a greatly reduced mortality compared with social classes IV and V (see 'all causes' in men and women). In specific causes of death, more variation occurs. In many, the disadvantage of social class V is very marked— mortality in this group is $2\frac{3}{4}$ times greater in cancer of the lung (men) and $3\frac{1}{2}$ times in cancer of the cervix uteri (women). However cancer of the breast (women) and suicide (women) show a different trend with social class I having the highest levels.

Table 2.13 Standardized Mortality Ratio by Cause and Social Class, England and Wales, 1970–72

Cause	Social Class					
	I	II	III N	III M	IV	V
All causes (men)	77	81	99	106	114	137
All causes (women)	82	87	92	115	119	135
Ischaemic heart disease (men)	88	91	114	107	108	111
Cancer of Lung (men)	53	68	84	118	123	143
Cancer of breast (women)	117	112	110	109	103	92
Cancer of cervix uteri	44	66	69	120	140	161
Suicide (women)	124	110	118	83	87	94

(From Occupational Mortality England and Wales 1970–72, OPCS)

Value of vital statistics

Each day in the wards, the nurse will constantly be concerned with various measurements to assess the health of the individual patient—taking temperatures, collection of specimens, assisting with biochemical or radiological investigations. She should look upon vital statistics in their various forms in the same way, for they represent the most reliable means available to measure the health of the community. No nurse need become an expert in vital statistics, but a simple knowledge and understanding of their uses will make her work more interesting. Community health problems change continuously and if the rudiments of the subject are understood, then the effects of these changes will mean so much more.

3
Maternal Health Services

In England and Wales about 656 000 births occur each year and the task of caring for the health of each mother is an important part of the health services.

Unlike almost any other speciality in medicine, the care of women in pregnancy is mainly a physiological one—there is nothing abnormal in the process itself. This has helped to create a very strong preventive service and the emphasis of all the maternity services is to avoid and prevent abnormalities occurring, and to recognize and diagnose them early so that if they do occur, their effects are minimized.

The maternity services are more closely co-ordinated than almost any other type of medical care. This is essential as the maternity service is shared between hospitals and the domiciliary services.

Hospital confinements

The proportion of mothers having their babies in hospitals varies with the area but in 1980 over all England 98.5 per cent had their confinements in hospital or nursing home and 1.5 per cent at home. However, there were many variations and many towns showed a hospital delivery rate over 99 per cent. The following are the groups of mothers who should *always be delivered in hospital*:

1　Those in whom there is an abnormality (such as toxaemia of pregnancy or malpresentation, e.g. breech).
2　Mothers with four or more children.
3　Mothers over the age of 35 years.
4　All *primigravidae* (mothers in their first pregnancy).
5　Mothers living in poor home conditions and for other serious social reasons.

There is an increasing tendency for mothers to be discharged during the first week following confinement. By 1980, 75 per cent of mothers delivered in hospital were discharged home on or before the 7th day of confinement.

The average stay in consultant maternity beds in hospital in England is 6.6 days and 4.7 days in general practitioner beds. The indications are that the tendency towards early discharge will be increased and some are discharged home as early as 48 hours after delivery. There are many social and domiciliary care problems created by such early discharge, for no mother is fit to look after her home at such an early stage of the puerperium and must have special help.

Administration of the Maternity Services

There is very strict control maintained over all maternity services by a central authority created for the purpose—the 'United Kingdom Central Council for Nursing, Midwifery and Health Visitors'. This body lays down rules for the conduct of all midwives. In addition, under the Midwives Acts, all unqualified persons, who are not either midwives or doctors (or students in training to become midwives or doctors), are prohibited from attending any woman in childbirth except to assist under the personal direction of a midwife or doctor, except in a sudden or urgent necessity. This rule prevents unskilled and untrained persons attending women in childbirth and so ensures indirectly that every woman is looked after by a fully-trained qualified person. The rules of the UK Central Council are supervised locally by the Regional Health Authority who usually delegates this responsibility to the District Health Authority. These rules include:

(a) Supervision over all certified midwives practising in the area. This covers midwives in maternity hospitals as well as those in nursing homes or employed as domiciliary midwives; in practice, the detailed supervision of midwives in maternity hospitals is left to the senior staff of those hospitals. The district health authority supervises midwives in nursing homes and domiciliary practice. No midwife may practise until she has given her notice to do so to the local supervising authority.

(b) Power to suspend a midwife from practice if it appears necessary to do so, to prevent spread of infection, e.g. it would be dangerous for a midwife who was a nasal carrier of pathogenic streptococci, to continue midwifery.

The UK Central Council itself lays down a code of practice and rules for all midwives. These specify the records she must keep, the standards she must follow in her midwifery practice, the drugs she may use, the anaesthetics she can use, as well as making it quite clear in what medical emergencies she has a duty to call in medical aid. In addition, the UK Central Council insists that every practising midwife shall attend a refresher course once every 5 years.

The rôle of general practitioner and midwife

If the mother is to be delivered at home there are three possibilities open to her:

1   In a minority of cases, her own general practitioner carries out the ante-natal care, delivers the patient and the midwife acts as a maternity nurse. Post-natal care also is undertaken by the general practitioner.
2   In most cases, the general practitioner does the ante-natal care but the midwife delivers the patient calling him only in case of need. The midwife reports delivery to the general practitioner who then completes the post-natal care.
3   She may choose to be delivered solely by a midwife who, in this instance, accepts full responsibility for looking after the patient in the ante-natal period and in her confinement.

In practice, it is usual for the mother to choose alternatives (1) or (2) as her own doctor is in an excellent position to help and advise his patient in the event of complications. General practitioners who have had special experience in midwifery and who undertake regular midwifery, are placed on the 'obstetric list'. They are then remunerated at a higher rate for each confinement than doctors who are not on the list.

Organization of a domiciliary midwifery service

Each District Health Authority employs the midwives who carry out the domiciliary work. At present there are very few private midwives.

The midwife can best be described as an expert practitioner of normal child bearing in all its varied aspects. At present, it is recommended that each midwife undertakes no more than 40 home deliveries a year if she is working on her own or 60 if she has, in addition, a pupil midwife assigned to her. She works very closely with the health visitor who should wherever possible be introduced to the mother during her ante-natal care (see page 57).

Each District Health Authority arranges an adequate midwifery coverage for the whole area. Often each midwife is provided with a house or flat from which to practise, and it is usual for her to have a car. This is particularly important as often she has to reach her patients quickly at any hour of the day or night, and to carry heavy equipment (including mobile gas and oxygen analgesia equipment).

Maternity outfits, which include all the necessary sterile dressings for the confinement and puerperium, are supplied free to each mother. It therefore is not necessary for the general practitioner to have to supply extra dressings for the confinement.

All midwives are trained in giving gas/oxygen analgesia. A medical certificate of fitness for analgesia must be obtained from the patient's own doctor during the pregnancy. Analgesia is available today to all mothers confined at home who wish to use it. Modern apparatus is very reliable and is designed to allow the patient to give herself (after tuition), her own gas/oxygen anaesthetic during the first stage of labour. The patient lies on her side, presses the mask with a pressure valve on it over her nose and breathes a mixture of gas and oxygen. As she loses consciousness, her grip relaxes, the mask falls away shutting off the valve and the supply of gas is cut off. She regains consciousness and may repeat the cycle if necessary.

Ante-natal care

The prevention of many complications of pregnancy rests more with careful ante-natal care than with any other factor. It is the responsibility of the midwife to ensure that adequate ante-natal care is carried out on her patients.

The mother due to be delivered in hospital usually receives ante-natal care by that hospital. Where this is difficult, arrangements are usually made for her to attend her own doctor for ante-natal care.

The pressure on most hospital ante-natal clinics is so great that it is not possible to carry out health education or mothercraft clinics in hospitals, and the usual arrangement is for the mothers to attend a special health education mothercraft clinic for this purpose. The first ante-natal examination usually takes place at the time of confirmation of the pregnancy, at about the third month of pregnancy.

A complete general medical examination must then be undertaken to ensure the woman has no undetected illness. At this time, a complete record should be obtained of past medical history paying particular attention to any past history of tuberculosis, diabetes and any virus infections from which the patient may have suffered. Chest X-rays are now only carried out if history or symptoms indicate that this would be wise.

The next stage is for a complete obstetric history to be taken of any previous pregnancies paying particular attention to any difficulties and abnormalities which may have occurred, either in her own or the baby's health. In all cases, blood tests should be taken and sent to the laboratory and include:

(a) A *Wassermann* or *Kahn* test to make certain that the mother *has no hidden infection of syphilis.* If it is found that she has a latent syphilitic infection at the third month of pregnancy and immediate treatment is started, *then a possible congenital infection in the infant can be avoided.*

(b) *Haemoglobin* estimation to check the level in each mother. If this is lower than normal, immediate treatment must be started. This is important as haemorrhage may occur later, and the results of such haemorrhage are bound to be more serious in cases where the haemoglobin level is lower than normal.

(c) *Blood Group* should be estimated and recorded. In an emergency, such information will be invaluable to enable a blood transfusion to be given quickly.

(d) *Rhesus factor* estimation should be carried out. If the mother is Rhesus positive then no problems will arise. If, however, the mother is Rhesus negative, difficulties may occur later affecting the health of her second and subsequent children. If the father is also Rhesus negative then all will be well. If, however, the father is Rhesus positive, which is more likely, then a further blood examination must be undertaken at the 34th week of pregnancy to check whether antibodies have developed in the mother's blood. If they have, then it is likely that the baby will develop serious haemolytic jaundice after birth and may need an exchange transfusion. For this reason, the patient must be delivered in hospital and the neighbouring paediatric unit should be alerted before the birth.

Even when antibodies are absent from a Rhesus negative mother's blood, blood from the baby's umbilical cord should be collected at birth and sent to a laboratory to be tested for antibodies.

Prevention of Rhesus incompatibility by immunization

It is now possible to prevent many of the problems of Rhesus incompatibility by immunization with Anti-D immunoglobulin of Rhesus negative women immediately after their first confinement or miscarriage. The problem in Rhesus incompatibility is due to red blood cells from a Rhesus positive child crossing the placental barrier and entering the mother's blood stream. Shortly after the birth of the first child, the Rhesus negative mother manufactures antibodies against these Rhesus positive red blood cells of her child which, in this way, are then destroyed. In second and subsequent pregnancies, these antibodies increase and, when they recross the placental barrier and enter the baby's blood stream, they lead to massive destruction of the baby's blood cells usually after birth, but in serious cases, before birth which may lead to a stillbirth.

Immunization with Anti-D immunoglobulin should be given *immediately following the first delivery* of a child or after *a first miscarriage or abortion*. An Anti-D immunoglobulin then destroys the Rhesus positive red blood cells of the baby within the mother's blood stream and there is not time enough for the mother to develop antibodies. Therefore a consequent pregnancy will be like a first pregnancy and no problems will arise. It is, however, necessary in such cases to *reimmunize the mother after all subsequent pregnancies or miscarriages to prevent antibody formation.*

Recommendations in regard to treatment are as follows:

1 In all cases the Anti-D immunoglobulin should be given within 60 hours of delivery or termination of pregnancy (miscarriage or abortion).

2 All Rhesus negative women giving birth to a Rhesus positive baby after the 20th week should be screened for fetal cells so that women who have large transplacental haemorrhages can be given large doses of Anti-D immunoglobulin.

3   The usual dose of Anti-D immunoglobulin for all Rhesus negative women having had Rhesus positive babies regardless of parity or ABO group, should initially be 100 μg. Further doses may be necessary for cases in which large transplacental haemorrhages have occurred.

4. A standard dose of 50 μg should be provided for all women known to be Rhesus negative, having therapeutic abortions up to and including the 20th week of pregnancy, except for those who are sterilized at the same operation. Rhesus negative women whose pregnancy with a Rhesus positive fetus is terminated after the 20th week should receive a dose of 100 μg.

5   The decision to use Anti-D immunoglobulin for Rhesus negative women having spontaneous abortions should be left to the individual clinician.

Dental care in pregnancy

Dental care in pregnancy is very important as the mother's teeth can deteriorate rapidly at this time. Every mother should, therefore, have a dental examination carried out immediately after the first ante-natal visit and arrangements made for any dental treatment needed to be done at once. Because care of the teeth is so important in pregnancy, special arrangements are made to treat, at no cost, all pregnant and nursing mothers (up to one year after confinement)—this free treatment includes the provision of dentures if needed. District Health Authorities arrange for this dental treatment to be carried out by their own dental staff at clinics.

Health education in pregnancy

The first ante-natal visit should be concluded by arranging for the mother to attend various health educational clinics to learn *mothercraft*. This is especially important to the mother having her first child (primipara) and gives her the opportunity to meet the health visitors who will help her after her baby's birth.

A visit should next be paid by the midwife or health visitor to the home. At this meeting, there should be frank discussion about many aspects of the pregnancy. Advice should especially be given concerning the diet for the mother.

Recent research has emphasized that there is a greater risk to the baby of a mother who smokes during pregnancy. In 1974 a health education campaign run by the Health Education Council spelt out these extra risks and pointed out that over 1500 babies annually might not have died if their mothers had given up smoking when they were pregnant. It also emphasized that smoking by the mother can lead to underweight at birth.

Prescription charges are waived to expectant mothers and until their baby is one year old. A Family Practitioner Committee Exemption certificate is needed; this is obtained by filling in Form FW8 obtainable from the doctor, midwife or health visitor.

Diet for pregnancy

A well-balanced diet with a good proportion of high-class protein is required. Many mothers have odd ideas about diet in pregnancy and the midwife must be patient and make certain that the diet required is fully understood. At least a pint of milk should be drunk per day and food-stuffs rich in iron, calcium, phosphorus and vitamins should be eaten. One or two eggs and a good helping of meat, fish, poultry or liver should be eaten per day. Cheese is also a most valuable food in pregnancy.

Vitamin preparations either in the form of tablets or orange juice and codliver oil may be obtained from the local clinic, or alternatively these may be taken in the diet by fresh fruit and various fats.

Good well-balanced meals will reduce the likelihood of unexplained prematurity and the incidence of toxaemia of pregnancy.

Maternity Grant and Allowance

These are dealt with in Chapter 18 (see page 280).

Free milk

An expectant mother with two or more children under school age is entitled to free milk, regardless of her family income.

Screening by amniocentesis

Amniocentesis is the removal, usually during the 16th week of pregnancy, of a small amount of amniotic fluid by means of a needle inserted through the uterine wall usually via the abdominal wall. This fluid can then be examined:

1 *microscopically*—the baby is surrounded by amniotic fluid in the uterus and a few cells will be cast off from the baby's skin and mucous membranes. These can be examined to give the chromosome pattern of the child (see Down's syndrome page 236).
2 *chemically* to estimate the level of alphafeta protein (AFP) which will, at 16 weeks of pregnancy, be raised in 99 per cent of cases of *open* neural tube defects.

In both instances, the object of carrying out the amniocentesis is to give an opportunity to the mother to have her pregnancy terminated by the 20th week if the results show that her baby is congenitally deformed. It is therefore most important that *counselling takes place before the 16th week*, and that *both parents fully understand the reasons for the investigation* and agree that, if the child is found to be abnormal, a termination of pregnancy should be carried out. If for any reason (religious or ethical) the parents would not agree to termination then this should be known before any tests are carried out for it is better that they should not be done at all.

Amniocentesis produces slight risks to the fetus. It is not easy to estimate these accurately but the most recent studies have indicated that there is approximately 1 per cent extra risk of fetal death. This is a maximum figure and is likely to be lower. There is also an increased possibility of respiratory difficulties in the fetus at birth and of orthopaedic postural deformities which may require immediate treatment. Because of this, after amniocentesis the birth should always take place in a maternity hospital with full paediatric support.

Screening tests to identify open neural tube defects

The following are the stages in the screening tests to identify open neural tube defects:

1 dating of the pregnancy accurately and counselling of the parents before the 16th week;
2 16th week – sample of mother's blood collected and alphafetaprotein (AFP) level estimated;
3 if AFP level is high repeat the test during 17th week;
4 if second test is also positive, carry out ultrascan (if this has not already been done), to check the duration of pregnancy and to exclude multiple pregnancy (twins);
5 undertake amniocentesis during 18th week and calculate the level of AFP in the amniotic fluid;
6 if raised, then the chance of the fetus having an open neural tube defect is very high (99 per cent) and an immediate termination of pregnancy should be carried out.

Counselling

Skilled counselling is essential, especially after a termination of pregnancy, to tell the parents:

(i) the nature of the malformation of the fetus;
(ii) the risks of a likely recurrence in another pregnancy.

After one abnormal pregnancy resulting in an open neural tube defect, the chance will be higher in a second (approximately 1 in 20); after two abnormal pregnancies, the risk rises to approximately 1 in 8. However, it is still possible to carry out the screening tests in further pregnancies and, if this is done, the risks of any abnormal child being born are minimal.

Screening to diagnose Down's syndrome

It is possible by amniocentesis to diagnose whether the fetus is suffering from Down's syndrome. It is advisable only to carry out amniocentesis where the risks of Down's syndrome *exceed* those to the fetus during the procedure of amniocentesis (approximately 1 per cent). This means in practice that amniocentesis to discover Down's syndrome should be carried out on pregnant women aged 36 and above. If all such mothers were screened in this way it has been estimated that the birth of about 18–20 per cent of babies with Down's syndrome could be prevented.

Continued ante-natal care

Further ante-natal examinations are regularly carried out during pregnancy— at least once a month until the 28th week and then every two weeks until the 36th week and, from that time until delivery, once a week. At each visit an abdominal examination is carried out. The position of the child is carefully observed and recorded during the last weeks of pregnancy and, particularly in the primipara, the *early engagement of the head in the pelvis* is checked. At each visit, the *blood pressure is examined*— it should never rise above 130/90 during pregnancy. In addition, the *urine is tested for albumin* and the legs palpated for oedema.

A careful *record is kept of the weight gain* during pregnancy, especially between the 20th and 30th weeks. If the weight gain exceeds 7 lbs (3.3 kg) in this period, especially in young primipara, this should be regarded as a sign of hypertensive disease of pregnancy. Such patients should be treated accordingly with a high-protein low-carbohydrate diet and observed very carefully at frequent intervals. If other signs of impending hypertensive disease of pregnancy develop, especially a raised blood pressure and or development of albuminuria, the patient should be given strict bed rest. She must be admitted to hospital for further treatment, if, in spite of bed rest, signs of toxaemia persist.

Value of ante-natal care in preventing serious abnormalities of pregnancy

It cannot be emphasized too strongly that good ante-natal care can reduce the dangers of serious abnormalities of pregnancy. Early in the ante-natal care programme of any mother, the possible danger of an ectopic pregnancy must be borne in mind. In 1979 ectopic pregnancy was the seventh commonest cause of maternal death and accounted for three deaths in England. Immediate operation is most important as soon as the diagnosis has been made. Resuscitation should not precede operation but be co-incidental with it.

The main dangers of hypertensive disease of pregnancy and haemorrhage can both be greatly reduced by careful ante-natal care. Any abnormality discovered in ante-natal work must be completely investigated. The following are a few of the more important ones:

(a) a raised blood pressure

(b) albuminuria

(c) oedema

(d) a loss of blood per vaginam even if this is only slight—a 'show'—may be a sign of placenta praevia

(e) the head of the child not fully engaging into the mother's pelvis. This is a very important factor in the primipara in whom the head should be fully engaged by the 36th week and often earlier. If the baby's head in the primipara is not engaged by this time, there is usually something wrong. Either the presentation is faulty, or there may be an abnormally small pelvis, which is rare today except in immigrant populations, or the pelvis may already contain the placenta—placenta praevia.

As the pregnancy nears its end regular ante-natal examinations become even more important. If a patient defaults from attending an ante-natal visit it is essential that the doctor or midwife call on her patient to find out the reason. In many instances, the reason may only be slackness on the part of the patient but it may be that she has developed some symptom which she does not recognize as serious but which gives her the excuse to postpone her visit. If such symptoms are the signs of an impending hypertensive disease of pregnancy, the midwife's visit may well be instrumental in ensuring that proper treatment is carried out promptly. This could make the difference between, in extreme cases, a live child plus healthy mother, or the tragedy of a maternal death with probably a stillbirth.

Puerperal phlebitis, thrombosis and pulmonary embolism make up the second commonest cause of maternal mortality. Its risk rises with age and parity of the mother and is increased by Caesarean section. It is important that the early signs of pulmonary embolism are not missed—not infrequently pleuritic pain is present but its significance is often not recognized and the patient is treated with antibiotics. In pregnancy such pain should always be treated seriously as it may indicate a pulmonary embolism.

Preventive aspects of maternal mortality

At present one mother per 8333 pregnancies loses her life as a result of childbearing. *Each maternal death is very carefully investigated to find the cause and whether there were any preventable factors in that death.* This enquiry is carried out by a consultant obstetrician and the community physician. The most recent series of such investigations collected together by the Department of Health and Social Security (1973–75) show that of present-day maternal deaths 59.6 per cent have some clear preventable factor. In other words, 59.6 per cent of the deaths caused by childbearing could have been avoided if some mistake or omission had not occurred. The types of 'preventable factors' vary from mistakes and omissions on the part of the doctors and midwives to lack of cooperation on the part of the patient herself.

When the great improvement over the last thirty-seven years in the safety of child bearing is examined (1 mother per 230 pregnancies died in 1936), it is easy to be complacent, but the fact remains that if all the preventable factors were reduced, and theoretically this is quite possible, only 1 in (approximately) 19 000 women would die, not 1 in 8333 as at present. Detailed examination of the types of mistake which lead to most of these deaths show that lack of adequate ante-natal care was the most important reason.

The eight most common causes of maternal mortality in the 1979 survey of maternal deaths in England and Wales were:

1	Complications of puerperium (including puerperal embolism)	21
2	Hypertensive disease of pregnancy (toxaemia)	13
3	Complications of labour and delivery	10
4	Abortion	9
5	Haemorrhage of pregnancy	8
6	Indications for care in pregnancy	5
7	Ectopic pregnancy	3
8	Other causes	5

Management of labour in domiciliary practice

Although only 1.5 per cent of births now occur at home, the following account is still given in detail as all home deliveries may present special hazards to the mother and child. Whether or not a doctor has been booked, usually the midwife is first notified when labour starts. She then visits the mother, examines her and if she confirms that labour has started, arranges for the care of the mother. The midwife will bring to each patient the anaesthetic apparatus plus all the equipment for the labour.

As explained earlier, the mother may give herself a whiff of anaesthetic either using gas and oxygen.

The midwife then reports to the doctor when labour has started. As most doctors have to carry on their busy practices, the midwife continues to look after the mother, only calling the doctor if some difficulty occurs.

A high degree of surgical cleanliness is maintained by using sterile gowns, masks, cap and sheets. Increasing use is being made of disposable sterile materials, and these now include towels, masks, caps and syringes. Any sterile gowns which are used remain at the patient's house to reduce any risk of carrying infection from patient to patient.

Midwives may leave the patient for a short time in the first stage of labour. They can give either pethidine or more commonly pethilorfin which has less depressant effect upon the child. Because labour often progresses rapidly after giving such drugs, no midwife should leave the patient after administering pethilorfin.

After delivery, the midwife may have to resuscitate the child. She has a special mucus sucker to clear the air passages of the child and also a sparklet oxygen resuscitator. This is a most valuable and neat apparatus which supplies oxygen at a measured rate for the baby to breathe and has made the problem of resuscitation much safer and surer.

If, during the labour, the midwife meets with any abnormality, she must send immediately for medical aid whilst staying herself to continue the delivery. Some District Health Authorities provide their midwives with portable radio transmitters so that they can summon medical aid without having to leave their patient. In most cases, medical aid will be provided by the doctor who is booked, but, if no doctor has been booked, the midwife sends for the nearest doctor who is on the obstetric list.

In more urgent and serious problems, the midwife may send for a special mobile hospital team, the 'flying squad'.

Use of hospital emergency team (flying squad)

Each maternity hospital has a mobile team (flying squad) consisting of an experienced obstetrician (consultant or registrar) plus an anaesthetist and an experienced hospital midwife, who will go to the home of a patient to deal with any emergency in labour. Usually such a team is taken to the patient's home by an ambulance. The most usual reasons for the flying squad to be sent for are:

1   *Sudden haemorrhage* (particularly post-partum haemorrhage). In this instance the flying squad helps to resuscitate the patient and for this purpose they carry blood and plasma for transfusion. They may also have to control bleeding and deal with its cause (say retained placenta). It is much safer to resuscitate the patient first and then move her to hospital.

2   *A complication of labour*—an example would be difficulty in the second stage of labour such as unexpected breech presentation.

Flying squads have proved themselves to be most valuable especially in large cities and one of their great assets is that they are readily available at all times. The general practitioner may be out on his rounds when help is urgently needed and it is reassuring to the midwife to know she can always obtain skilled help by calling out the flying squad.

The flying squad is called out to 1 in approximately 70 domiciliary births—the causes being for haemorrhage in a third of the cases, for retained placenta in half the cases and for varying difficulties in the remainder.

The cooperation card

Although domiciliary midwifery usually does not involve the hospital service, cooperation, as shown by the value of the flying squad, is of great importance. Cooperation between services is helped by every woman whether booked to have her baby in hospital or at home *always carrying a special cooperation card with her*. This is a simple record of her ante-natal care, containing all the information which is invaluable in an emergency. If a patient booked for home confinement suddenly requires, urgent hospital admission, this cooperation card is of great value in arranging for prompt and proper treatment. It records the results of all tests carried out including blood group, and can therefore save valuable time.

Post-natal care

Six weeks after delivery a full post-natal examination should be carried out either at the hospital where the baby was born or at the doctor's surgery or at the clinic. By this time the health visitor should be acting as one of the most important advisors to the mother (see Chapter 4).

Care of the unmarried mother

The care of the unmarried mother in pregnancy is a special problem and approximately 11.8 per cent of all births occur in mothers who are unmarried. Illegitimacy produces many difficulties and, from the preventive health point of view, the most serious immediate problem is that the social circumstances surrounding an unmarried mother produce greater hazards to both mother and child. These are mainly connected with the fact that no ante-natal care may be carried out because of concealment of the pregnancy, or the mother may be forced to leave her home due to unsympathetic parental reaction. The extra hazard to the baby in an illegitimate birth is shown quite dramatically in an increased infant mortality rate of 21 for illegitimate births compared with a rate of 10 for legitimate births.

Wherever possible, arrangements are made to help the unmarried mother to stay at home. If the rift so often created between parents and the mother-to-be can be healed, problems tend to be reduced and hospital delivery and possible early adoption may provide the best result possible.

In about half of the cases, however, the unmarried mother cannot and does not wish to stay at home. In such instances the best solution is for her to be helped by a social services department who can usually arrange a suitable hostel or similar unit, many of which are run by church or voluntary organisations. After the birth of the child in hospital many unmarried mothers need time to decide whether they wish to care for the child or arrange adoption. An increasing number now care for their children and are accommodated in flats or sheltered housing.

Sheltered housing for unmarried mothers

Independent accommodation for the unmarried mother where she can live with her baby for $1\frac{1}{2}$–2 years after confinement has been introduced in a few areas and has proved very successful. By using day nursery services the mother is able to go out to work and lead a more normal independent life than is possible in hostels. Late permanent housing is often arranged and with the help of a day nursery run by the social services department the mother can undertake a full-time job.

German measles and pregnancy

An attack of german measles (rubella) during the first three months of pregnancy can result in harmful effects to the fetus. These include a higher proportion of abortion and stillbirths and an increased incidence of congenital abnormalities, especially congenital cataract in the child, congenital heart disease or deafness. Research has also shown a much higher infant mortality in children of mothers who develop rubella during the first three months of pregnancy. Active immunization is advocated for all girls aged 11–13 years (see page 91). Vaccination of women of child-bearing age is not recommended routinely. If an adult woman wishes vaccination, a serological test, which can be carried out by the Public Health Laboratory Service should always be undertaken. Vaccination should only be offered to those who are seronegative (approximately 10 per cent of adult women without a history of rubella). *It is most important that a woman is not pregnant at the time of the vaccination, and does not become pregnant for at least two months after protection.*

Any mother who has never had german measles or has not been immunized and who comes into contact with the disease during the first three months of pregnancy should be promptly *immunized with immunoglobulin*. This normally prevents an attack of german measles developing and protection lasts for six weeks and so avoids subsequent congenital deformities in the child.

It is, however, essential to realize that any danger from german measles *only occurs within the first three/four months of pregnancy* and that a later attack does no harm. Therefore, reassurance is often needed when this occurs.

Family planning

Under the National Health Service (Family Planning) Act, 1967, District Health Authorities have power to provide family planning advice together with the issue of contraceptive substances and appliances *on medical and social grounds*.

The National Health Service (Family Planning Amendment) Act, 1972, placed vasectomy on the same basis as other contraceptive services which the District Health Authority may provide. Before vasectomy is undertaken there should be:

1 counselling by a doctor experienced in family planning before operation.
2 adequate facilities for operation (including access to inpatient beds should a complication arise).
3 adequate follow-up including an alternative method of contraception *until a negative semen has been obtained on two occasions at an interval of one month.*

Family planning services are based on three important principles:

1 Comprehensive family planning advice should be available free of charge to all who wish to have it. It is hoped to increase clinic provision and more advice will be given to maternity and abortion patients. The domiciliary service is very important and arrangements are made to give such advice in the patient's own home if it is unlikely that she will attend a clinic.
2 General health education should include information on family planning.
3 Free contraceptive supplies should be available for those who need them (with the exception of the condom). This category includes those with a special social need who would otherwise be unlikely to undertake effective contraception and those with a financial need.

All other people, including those with a *medical need* for family planning, pay the standard prescription charge.

General practitioners also have a very important rôle in family planning and such advice should be offered by general practitioners and health visitors without waiting for people to ask for it. General practitioners can prescribe contraceptive pills on prescription forms EC 10. (Recent advice from the Committee on Safety of Drugs has emphasized that oral contraceptives with a low oestrogen, 20–50 mcg, were associated with a lower incidence of thrombo-embolic complications than earlier pills).

Recently, health authorities have developed a special domiciliary family planning service for women who suffer from ill health, live in poor social circumstances and are overburdened with too many children and who do not find it easy to attend a clinic. Southampton and York pioneered this service which is now being started in other areas. Such domiciliary family planning services have been shown to be of great value in helping to prevent deterioration in such problem families.

The methods of contraception used in England and Wales by persons attending family planning clinics in 1978 were:

	Thousands
Oral contraception	847.9
Intrauterine device	295.8
Sheath	128.9
Cap/Diaphragm	113.2
Vasectomy	16.2
'Chemical' methods	13.7
Sterilization	1.3
Rhythm method	0.2

Abortion

Since the introduction of the Abortion Act, 1967, abortion is legal in the United Kingdom where it can be shown by two doctors that the physical or mental health of the mother or children would be seriously affected by the birth.

The abortion (except in an emergency) must be performed in a National Health Service hospital, in one of the approved services hospitals, or in a place for the time being approved by the Secretary of State for the purposes of the Act.

The details of the present law are capable of considerable variations of interpretation; pregnancy may be terminated by a doctor if two registered medical practitioners are of the opnion, formed in good faith:

(a) that the continuance of the pregnancy would involve risk of the life of the pregnant woman or of injury to the physical or mental health of the pregnant woman or any existing children of her family, greater than if the pregnancy were terminated, or

(b) that there is a substantial risk that if the child were born it would suffer from such physical or mental abnormalities as to be seriously handicapped.

In assessing (a) account may be taken of the pregnant woman's actual or reasonably foreseeable environment.

Nursing homes undertaking abortion and pregnancy advice bureaux have to be approved by the Secretary of State and by the end of 1978, 34 such centres and 61 nursing homes had been approved.

4
Preventive Child Health Services

Care in the neo-natal period (birth to 28 days)

The first month of any child's life, the neo-natal period, is one of the most critical, for it is then that the majority of infant deaths occur. In 1982 the rate of infant deaths under one year per 1000 live births was 10.8 but 6.3 was the rate for deaths in the first month (neo-natal mortality).

It is, therefore, very essential that great care is taken with the newborn child.

Haemolytic disease of the newborn (see also pages 40–41)

Cases which are not immunized with Anti-D immunoglobulin. At birth every baby of a Rhesus negative mother should have some blood removed from the umbilical cord to test for antibodies which, if present, will gradually destroy the baby's red blood corpuscles by haemolysis. If the blood test shows antibodies to be present, the baby must be immediately admitted to hospital for treatment. This may include an exchange blood transfusion, which sets out to dilute continuously the antibodies and thus reduces the danger of blood destruction.

A simple perspex device for estimating the depth of jaundice in a newborn child (an icterometer) should be carried by every midwife and is useful to help judge the depth of any jaundice. It is especially useful to record the intensity of jaundice in premature babies.

Neo-natal cold injury

Although the very small premature baby is liable to suffer from chilling, it is now recognized that this is also a hazard in normal children. If any baby in its first month of life becomes seriously chilled, its body temperature may fall dangerously low to 32.2°C (90°F) or lower. The baby then becomes quiet and difficult to rouse and feed, and is cold to touch, and later oedematous. It may have a deceptively florid red complexion.

The prevention of this condition involves making certain that the temperature of the room in which the baby is sleeping does not fall below 18°C (65°F). Each midwife has a wall thermometer which should be left near the baby's cot to record the present temperature and the minimum temperature. This check and control is most important in winter but is still needed in summer, when unexpectedly low air temperatures may occur at night.

Care of the low birth weight baby

The majority of illnesses and death occur in babies of low birth weight (premature babies). As it is never possible to say with complete accuracy the length of any pregnancy, a baby whose birth weight is less than 2500 g (5½ lbs) is classified as needing special care. Approximately 6.8 per cent of all babies come into this category.

The chance of survival falls rapidly as the birth weight of the baby falls. With babies between 2250 g (5 lbs) and 2500 g (5½ lbs) birth weight 1.2 per cent die within 28 days but, for premature babies whose birth weight is under 1500 g (3½ lbs) 39 per cent die within 28 days.

The special hazards for a low birth weight baby child is shown by the neo-natal death rate (deaths within first 28 days of life) for such children is 8–9 times greater than for all children.

The reduction of mortality from prematurity can be achieved in two ways:

(a) by avoiding prematurity
(b) by improving care facilities for premature babies when born.

Avoidance of low birth weight babies

In many instances the exact cause of low birth weight is unknown. However, in some cases it will be associated with severe hypertensive disease of pregnancy, and first-class ante-natal care which reduces the incidence of this condition will also lessen the risk of it occurring.

Another important cause is chronic malnutrition in the mother and this is why the diet of each mother in pregnancy should be carefully watched. Generally, poor living conditions, overwork and increased frequency of infection, are also associated with a larger incidence of low birth weight babies. There is a greater frequency in women from Social Class IV and V (unskilled labourers, etc.) than in Social Class I and II. Improvements in living conditions will help reduce its incidence.

Care of low birth weight babies

It is convenient to subdivide all premature babies into two groups—those under 2000 g (4½ lbs) and who should be admitted to a special intensive care unit, while the second group, from 2000 g (4½ lbs) to 2500 g (5½ lbs), can be looked after at home, provided the home is satisfactory and there is a special domiciliary nursing service.

Intensive care units for low birth weight babies

Special intensive care units for low birth weight babies should be provided in all large maternity departments. Such units are usually designed to look after a small number of such infants. The care of the very small premature baby calls for skilled nursing using many modern techniques.

Incubator care will be needed for the very small premature babies. The value of the incubator is that it makes it easier to control the atmosphere in which the baby lives. There are three main factors:

1 The *temperature* of the incubator should be maintained so that the baby's temperature is kept *constant* at just below 36.6°C (98°F).
2 There should also be a *constancy* in the *relative humidity* within the incubator. It is best to keep the relative humidity (level of water vapour in the air) constantly at 60 per cent.
3 The *supply of oxygen* should be controlled. As many premature babies have difficulties in pulmonary ventilation (they often develop hyaline membrane disease after birth) oxygen can be most helpful, but *great care must be taken not to increase the level of oxygen too high*, for if this is done, there is danger of damaging the retina of the new-born child and producing blindness (retrolental fibroplasia). Thus, the level of oxygen is always kept at the lowest which will give adequate relief to the child.

Feeding

There are many different methods of feeding used. Because of the effort of sucking, breast feeding is rarely possible for very tiny babies. But human breast milk may be used from a human *breast milk bank* which is usually set up at the largest paediatric centres. Various forms of artificial feeding are used—often carefully graduated weaker feeds of dried milks. These are always given more frequently than usual, two or three hourly, and often given by nasal catheter, allowing the measured feed to flow by gravity.

Prevention of infection

To all very small babies, *infections* represent their greatest hazard. The development of a respiratory infection in a small premature baby may be so sudden and dramatic that death may result after a few hours. The prevention of infection is, therefore, one of the most important tasks of the nurses in charge of a premature baby unit. Strict rules must always be observed. No one (other than the parents) should enter an intensive care unit unless his presence is essential. No one should enter if suffering from an infection (cold or upper respiratory infection). Everyone must wear sterile cap, mask and gown. Hand washing must be scrupulously carried out.

Great care must be taken not to carry infection from one cot to another and very high nursing standards are essential. New admissions, especially if admitted from home, should be separated from those already being nursed within the unit.

In some units, air sterilization is practised using ultra-violet light filters.

Prevention of hypoxia and cerebral palsy

There is increasing evidence that low levels of oxygen in a baby's bloodstream (hypoxia) can damage the brain. This is most likely to occur with the low weight baby and can produce cerebral palsy. This damage can occur either late in pregnancy, due to death of part of the placenta, or in the first few days after the birth. Continuous monitoring of the level of oxygen in the baby's bloodstream, which is now possible in the best intensive care units, has been shown to reduce the incidence of cerebral palsy by 35–40 per cent. Although such preventive treatment is only possible in certain centres, it is hoped to extend its use in the future.

Domiciliary care of low birth weight babies

The larger low birth weight babies, between 2000 g ($4\frac{1}{2}$ lbs) and 2500 g ($5\frac{1}{2}$ lbs) weight, can be looked after quite adequately at home provided the home is reasonable and that there is a special *domiciliary nursing baby service*. This is run by the District Health Authority and consists of specially trained nurses, who may also be midwives, whose task it is to look after the small baby at home. The nurse has special equipment such as cots, feeding equipment and thermometers, which can be loaned to the mother. The nurse then teaches the mother all the necessary information especially about feeding problems, and follows this up by daily or twice-daily visits to each baby, to ensure that care is continuing properly. In this way, continuous advisory help is available to the mothers and it also ensures that, if any difficulty or illness occurs, it can be promptly treated. In many cases ignorance plays a large part in producing problems in the low birth weight baby looked after at home. The great value of domiciliary nursing baby service is that it reduces the effects of such ignorance.

The nurses who staff the service must do nothing else and must be careful to avoid introducing infection within the home. Visitors to the baby must be as carefully controlled as in hospital. In practice, infection is not as large a problem in the domiciliary service as in the hospital intensive care unit as there is much less danger of cross infection from other patients and staff, as the human contacts with the baby at home are so limited.

Care of the normal baby

Rôle of the Health Visitor in home care

The standard of care and help given to the mother within a month after her confinement in helping with the care of her child is most important. It is during this period that the basis of sound health in the child can be formed.

The care of the child immediately after birth will be by the staff of the maternity ward, if a hospital birth, or by the midwife who delivered the baby, if the birth took place at home. When the mother leaves hospital after delivery, the midwife will take over the care of the baby for a few days. After the 14th day, the main adviser to the mother, apart from the family doctor who is usually only consulted if some illness or extreme difficulty occurs, is the *health visitor.*

The health visitor is a highly trained nurse who, after gaining an SRN qualification and attending an obstetrics course, must then attend a year's full-time course in social and preventive medicine and qualify by examination for a Health Visitor's Certificate. The main task of the health visitor is to ensure that all the family and especially the children are as healthy as possible. This is achieved by a continuous process of health education and the health visitor strives to become the welcomed adviser to the mother and family in all health matters.

If possible, the health visitor meets the mother during her pregnancy at mothercraft classes so that she gets to know her. She takes over from the midwife the responsibility of the mother and child at the 14th day after delivery. It is best if this can be done by the midwife and health visitor meeting at the mother's home on the 14th day. Increasingly it is becoming usual for the link up between the general practititioner and health visitor to be closer and closer and so the health visitor today will usually be working in the primary health care team with the general practitioner who is also in charge of the patient.

Infant feeding

The first important factor upon which the health visitor concentrates is the feeding of the child. Wherever possible, breast feeding is recommended. To establish breast feeding much patience and encouragement are needed. The temptation to give up the effort because of difficulties is often great and much anxiety is felt by mothers who fear the baby is not getting enough milk on the breast.

A national committee recently looked into present day practice in infant feeding and unanimously agreed that the best food for babies is human breast milk, and that, when successfully managed, breast feeding of four to six months duration offers many advantages to both mother and infant. Since the risks of ill health are greater when the baby is very young, breast feeding for even as short a period as two weeks is an advantage.

It is difficult to be certain of the proportion of babies that are breast fed today. Recent investigations have shown much variation but the proportion is about 25 per cent of all children at 4 months. The increased tendency for some mothers to return to work after two months, and the ease and convenience of artificial feeding have tended to reduce breast feeding. It is, however, important to realize that the infant who is breast fed for five to six months has the best possible start in life. There is a lot of evidence that the incidence of all types of infection is lowest in breast fed children. In outbreaks of infantile gastroenteritis, which can be a dangerous disease in young infants, the breast fed child almost invariably escapes. There is also evidence that the personal bond between mother and child is never closer than between the mother and her child whom she has breast fed.

Health visitors therefore do all they can to encourage breast feeding. If, however, this is not possible, then the health visitor constantly helps the mother by giving her advice regarding artificial feeding. Today the majority of artificial feeding is by use of dried milks which are reconstituted just before the baby's feed. There are many different kinds. Suitable dried milks are available at health authority maternity and child health clinics at low cost. It is also usual to sell other proprietary baby foods at such clinics.

The health visitor also advises and helps the mother with all the small day-to-day problems of bringing up a baby. Frequency of feeding, clothing to be used, room temperature, general hygiene and the sleep patterns of babies, are all dealt with. A most important aspect of a health visitor's work is that she visits the home of the mother and there can give practical advice and health education in the mother's own environment, which the mother herself will have to use. She can make certain the mother fully understands all the intricacies attached to caring for a small baby. Each health visitor hopes that the mother will look forward to her visits as those of a friend and adviser.

Child health clinics

By the end of the first month, it is expected that the feeding of the baby will be progressing satisfactorily and the mother is invited to bring her baby along to the nearest child health clinic.

The child health clinic is the local headquarters of the preventive medical services for children and is designed as a place to which the mother can bring her baby at any time for help and advice. No ill child should ever be taken to such a clinic but should be seen by the general practitioner. In cases of doubt, the health visitor will call to see the baby at home. It is important to avoid bringing ill babies to child health clinics because of the risk of spreading infection.

Each child health clinic is staffed by the same health visitors who do the home visiting in the area. The functions of the clinic include:

(a) *Education in mothercraft*—this is carried out by individual tuition to mothers or group tuition with help of leaflets, posters, lectures and films. All health education topics are discussed, including the avoidance of accidents in the home.

(b) *Sale of infant foods* including:
  (i) Suitable dried milks
  (ii) Vitamin drops for infants
  (iii) Vitamin tablets for expectant and nursing mothers (these also contain calcium, phosphate and iodine)
  (iv) Certain other baby foods.

Mixed feeding in infants usually starts any time between 12 and 15 weeks. There is a wide variety of special baby foods now available which are usually sold in tins or jars and are made up from many types of strained baby foods made from many meats and vegetables. There are also many different cereals available so that any baby now gets used to a wide variety of new tastes.

(c) *Routine medical inspection*—A doctor attends the clinic and sees the mother and examines her child on the first visit and usually at three months, six months and one year, and subsequently annually. The doctor is also available if the health visitor or mother wishes to see him in between their routine examinations, the purpose of which is to check that the baby is perfectly fit and to discover any abnormalities as soon as possible.

(d) *To give advice on minor problems* as they arise. Much of this will be done by the health visitor during home visits but mothers are also encouraged to visit the clinic if they have problems in between home visits. Feeding problems and difficulties connected with the development of the child are usual reasons for such visits.

(e) *To give protective immunizations to infants*. These immunizations, which can also be given by the general practitioner in his surgery, are fully discussed in Chapter 6 and include immunization against whooping cough, diphtheria, tetanus, measles, poliomyelitis and, in girls, rubella.

Screening tests to discover unsuspected illness

During the first few months of a baby's life, it is important to carry out various checks on the health of the child to make certain that all abnormalities are spotted (such tests are called 'screening' tests).

Phenylketonuria

This is a rare metabolic disease (incidence approximately 1 in 10 000) in which the metabolism of the infant is faulty and poisonous phenylalanine metabolites are produced which eventually lead to a marked retarded mental development, and the child develops severe mental handicap. If treatment is started when first symptoms of mental handicap show themselves, it is too late. However, if the disease can be diagnosed within a few weeks of birth, and the child given a special diet, this mental deterioration can be avoided.

Every child has a simple blood test—the Guthrie test—carried out on a specimen of blood taken from the baby between the sixth and fourteenth day of life. Several spots of blood from the young infant are collected from a heel prick on to specially absorbent filter paper. In the laboratory a small disc is punched out of each of the blood-impregnated filter papers and up to 100 individual discs are placed on a special agar plate containing a spore suspension of *Bacillus subtilis*, and an inhibitory substance Phenylalanase acts as an antagonist to the inhibitor; after incubation in positive tests growth of the organism will be observed around the blood disc.

At present about 95 per cent of babies born in the United Kingdom are tested for phenylketonuria.

Neo-natal hypothyroidism

It is now possible to screen new born babies for hypothyroidism which, if undetected, can lead to permanent brain damage within a few months and to mild to severe mental handicap. The incidence of neo-natal hypothyroidism is about 1 in 5000. Provided the condition is recognized and treated before the 3rd month of life, 74 per cent achieve an IQ of 90 or greater whereas if the diagnosis is delayed until the 4th to 6th month, only 33 per cent come into this category. The test involves measuring by radio immuno assay, the thyroid hormone (T4) or the Thyroid Stimulating Hormone (TSH) of the pituitary in the baby's blood. The TSH test is more specific and is always used to make the final diagnosis, but the advantage of the T4 test is that the blood collected for the phenylketonuria test can be used for both. It is therefore cheap and relatively easy to introduce. It is hoped that screening will be widely introduced throughout the UK in the next few years. With widespread screening for neo-natal hypothyroidism, it has been estimated that 150 infants a year could be prevented from developing brain damage and mental handicap.

Congenital dislocation of the hip

Another good example of a condition which, if diagnosed very early, can be quite simply and completely treated but which, if diagnosed later, is difficult to treat and may lead to permanent disability, is *congenital dislocation of the hip*.

It is now known that the main cause of this condition is inadequate development of the acetabulum of the pelvis.

There is a simple test (eliciting Ortolani's or von Rosen's sign) which the midwife or health visitor should carry out on all babies at birth and at monthly intervals until the child is 4 months old. In this test, the hip of the child is manipulated from the adducted to the abducted position while the thigh is flexed. A positive result is indicated by a 'click' or 'snap' being produced during the test and corresponds with the dislocated femoral head moving into the proper position in the acetabulum.

If the test is abnormal, the child should be referred without delay to an orthopaedic surgeon. Treatment is simple and consists of maintaining the hips continuously in abduction until the subluxation has been corrected. The constant pressure of the head of the femur in the centre of the acetabulum causes it to deepen and develop normally. After treatment for six to nine months, the danger to the infant of congenital dislocation of the hip disappears.

Screening for deafness

The recognitition of congenital deafness is difficult and depends on careful observation of the infant during the first eight months of life, and on recognizing the different vocalization patterns in the normal and deaf child from 3 to 8 months of age. Both develop in the same way until 3 months old, making reflex sounds and responding to a *loud* noise. But from 3 months onwards, the deaf child's vocalization diminishes steadily so that by 8 months, little effort is made to produce sounds, although the child will still remain alert, attentive and interested in its surroundings. By comparison, the normal child increases his sounds which become more tuneful, and is clearly copying what is heard. This changing pattern in the deaf child is often more easily recognized by the health visitor who plays an important part in diagnosing congenital deafness.

Importance of follow-up of certain infants

Although screening for congenital abnormalities is now undertaken on all infants by doctors and health visitors, a high proportion are found in children in whom:

1   *Family history* is suggestive of—
    Any deafness, blindness or cerebral palsy
    Any known congenital abnormalities
    Mental disorder

2 *Obstetric history* is abnormal. These include any illness or abnormality of the mother in pregnancy—rubella, excessive vomiting, threatened abortion, toxaemia, multiple pregnancy, premature birth, asphyxia, prolonged labour.
3 *Post-natal problems* occur, including difficulties in sucking, convulsions or any serious illness in the first few months of life.

For all children coming within this group, special attention should be paid during the first five years of life and their follow-up is the responsibility not only of the health visitor but also the general practitioner and paediatric departments.

Cot deaths (sudden infant deaths)

The sudden infant death syndrome—often called 'cot death'—is a very distressing event, for such a death occurs very suddenly and unexpectedly. The aetiology of the condition is not fully known but it is now recognized that there is not one simple cause. In approximately one-third of all cases, a known disease capable of causing the death is present; in another third, minimal signs of disease are found which, although unlikely to cause the death, may contribute to it. In the remaining instances, although recognized disease is absent, there is evidence of disturbed growth. *Sudden death in a completely well infant or in one which is being breast fed is very rare.*

Many cases occur in infants in social class IV and V or in families with special social problems. More occur in 'inner city' or disadvantaged areas and the reduction of such deaths may be more connected with better health visiting and more effective primary health care to such deprived areas. Prevention, in the present stage of knowledge, is inexact but studies in Sheffield suggest that it may be possible to identify families whose children may be at potential risk. Such families need more concentrated antenatal and postnatal care and health education and support from health visitors and services in such areas should be structured to enable this to occur.

Care of normal children, 6 months to 5 years of age

The preventive care of children from six months to five years of age continues along similar lines. Periodic visits are made to the child's home and his progress is checked from time to time at the child health clinic or by visits to his own doctor. The two approaches which are followed are:

(a) checking that normal progress is being maintained,
(b) complete investigation of any illness or abnormality discovered.

Normal stages of development in children

Normal progress in any child is checked by watching the various stages of growth reached, and checking that these are not late in appearing. The normal baby should be able to sit with support by the 3rd or 4th month and by the 7th to sit alone. By the 8th or 9th month standing should be possible with support and without support between the 10th and 14th months. Walking will follow shortly after the infant can stand without support. Crawling or creeping usually occurs about the 9th or 10th month but may not always be shown.

In the past, probably too much attention was paid to a baby's weight as indicating progress. It is still useful in indicating change in progress—a sudden loss of weight or halting in the gain in weight always calls for further investigation. However, no reliance should be placed on tables giving 'normal' weights for children of different ages due to the wide variations commonly seen in normal children.

Usually a *baby will double his birth weight by 5 months and treble it by 12 months*. Sudden changes in weight, e.g. suddenly ceasing to gain weight, are indicators for further investigation. There is much individual variation. In particular, care must be taken not to stress to the mother too much the baby's weight, for it should never be her main guide to his progress. It is interesting to note that some of the fittest babies who have been breast fed are often lighter than average but are very active and alert.

The general behaviour of the child is also an important guide—he should be a happy active child who constantly explores the home in an inquisitive way. It is most important that the child always feels secure.

Sphincter control of the bladder is slow to develop. It usually does so at the end of the first year and may not be completely reliable until the child is $2\frac{1}{2}$ to 3 years old. It is important that the mother realizes this for futile attempts to train the baby too young may only cause undue irritation and tensions, and may later produce the opposite effect in enuresis. These and other problems should be freely discussed between the mother and health visitor and, in this way, most of the difficulties will be avoided.

Weaning from either breast milk or from bottled feeds commences between three and six months of age. Today, with the many specially prepared foods for weaning (including tinned foods), this is simple. In many clinics, such foods are sold and the health visitor is always there to advise on their use.

The development of speech in a child is a very important stage. The first primitive efforts to produce speech start at 7 or 8 months of age. The child begins to imitate what he hears and to associate people and objects with the sounds he makes. By $1\frac{1}{2}$ years of age, he should be using simple words and simple sentences.

A very slow development of speech should always lead to a careful re-testing of hearing. The completely deaf child hears nothing to imitate and, unless taught by special methods, will never speak. The other important reason for severe retardation of speech is lack of normal mental development. Further examination in such a case will show retardation in other stages of physical development.

Clothing and shoes

As the child begins to walk, it is most important that his clothing and shoes always fit. Many crippling deformities of the feet have been produced by ill-fitting shoes at all ages. As far as possible, shoes with wide fitting toes should be selected. It is also important to make certain that the child's socks are the correct size. If they have shrunk and are too short, they will exert constant pressure on the toes and may lead to overlapping of toes and other deformities. Because no two children have similar shaped feet, it is always wise not to pass on shoes to younger children in the same family. This can, however, be safely done for loose fitting footwear such as wellington boots.

A constant watch should be kept on the way in which the feet of the toddler are developing. Minor deformities such as flat feet, pes cavus and rigid feet can be spotted easily. All respond much more readily to treatment at this age than later. Early diagnosis can thus do much to prevent subsequent problems.

Intestinal infestations

Minor infestations with *threadworms* are quite commonly seen at this age. The worms often migrate from the rectum to the buttocks at night time leading to much itching and irritation. This is often the cause of toddlers sleeping fitfully. Diagnosis is easy—examination of the anus shows the tiny migrating worms. Once diagnosed, treatment with modern drugs is easy using piperazine phosphates, and prevents further problems.

Safety of young children

As the child grows up, he becomes more and more inquisitive and thus may become liable to accidents and illnesses.

In Great Britain, about 250 children die each year as a result of accidents in the home. Over 4000 children aged 0–4 are admitted to hospital for burns and scalds and a hundred under 5 die, but many more are left with scarring and have to face recurrent admissions to hospital for skin grafting.

Climate

Excessive heat or cold can be dangerous (see also page 53 for neo-natal cold injury). Older babies can also be affected to a lesser degree; no infant should go out of doors in very cold or foggy weather. Babies also ought to avoid intense heat and a pram can become a heat trap. The hood should be kept down in sunny weather and a sun canopy should be used. Under no circumstances should a baby be left in an unventilated car in summertime.

Prams

The brake must be tested regularly. Cat nets must be used as a cat may snuggle against a baby's face for warmth and suffocate him. A baby harness should be used later in a pram for all infants sitting up.

Cots and bedding

Pillows are unnecessary and dangerous to young babies for their use may lead to suffocation. Under no circumstances should a cot be painted with a lead based paint as the child may later suck the sides of the cot and be poisoned.

Feeding

It is possible for a baby to choke on a bottle propped up in a cot or pram. No baby should ever be left alone with a bottle and all feeding must be carefully supervised.

Prevention of home accidents

The most common accidents include:

1 Inhalation of food or other objects leading to obstruction and suffocation
2 Mechanical suffocation
3 Fire
4 Falls
5 Poisoning.

Each year many children under 5 years of age die as a result of such accidents in the home. All are preventable and continual efforts are made by health visitors to reduce these casualties. Mothers are taught the dangers of letting young children play with unsuitable objects such as plastic bags, the importance of fireguards and flameproof clothing, the dangers of unprotected stairs and of brightly coloured medical tablets, many of which are poisonous to young children and which look so like sweets to them.

Some District Health Authorities have introduced a special loan scheme for fireguards and all are constantly engaged in health education efforts to reduce the needless loss of life and invalidism caused by these tragic home accidents.

Care of acute illness in the child aged 1 to 5 years

In families, it is not unusual for the younger children to become infected with the common childhood infectious diseases, such as measles, whooping cough, scarlet fever. Treatment is similar to that for older children but it is always important to remember that such illnesses may be the starting point for various chronic minor inflammatory and catarrhal conditions such as tonsillitis, sinusitis, or otitis media. With modern chemotherapy and antibiotic treatment many of the serious chronic conditions such as otitis media can be avoided *provided that early diagnosis is made and treatment started*. It is important that such acute infections in children are treated promptly.

The treatment of the child with enlarged tonsils depends:

(i) on whether the child has successive attacks of tonsillitis;
(ii) whether there is associated respiratory obstruction from enlarged and inflamed adenoids;
(iii) whether infection spreads to involve the ear.

If any of the above three are present, tonsillectomy should be carried out as soon as the child is well again. Prompt removal of the adenoids in such children is likely to prevent serious otitis media. Tonsils today are rarely removed just because they are enlarged.

Various squints may become obvious in this age group and the doctor or health visitor should always check if there is any sign of such defects. Early diagnosis and effective treatment will do much to reduce the likelihood of chronic and serious problems later.

Congenital malformations

Congenital malformations are notifiable by District Health Authorities to the Office of Population Censuses and Surveys. Pre-natal infections such as rubella or the use of certain drugs in early pregnancy such as thalidomide can cause congenital abnormalities and it is hoped that by careful continuous analysis any increase would be noticed more quickly. Just under 13 000 babies in England and Wales are born with congenital abnormalities each year. Approximately 8.35 per cent of children have one, 12.5 per cent two, 3 per cent three and 1 per cent four or more malformations. The age and parity of the mother are factors in determining the levels of incidence: the lowest rates are in the younger mothers having their second child, while the highest rates are in mothers over 40 having their fourth child.

Talipes is the commonest malformation followed by spina bifida, cleft lip or palate, congenital dislocation of the hip and Down's syndrome. Boys show more abnormalities than girls (5:4), but this is mainly due to external genital abnormalities.

Coordination of child health services and education and social services

At all times, it is essential to ensure coordination between the child health services and the education and social services. Health visitors and social workers should work closely together (see page 57) and both should undertake domiciliary care for children who are either handicapped or have special problems.

In many handicapped children, the special education (see page 77) which they need should start before 2 years of age. Such children when they reach the age of 17 years will become the responsibility of the social services, although all education authorities continue to have some responsibility as regards continuing education until they reach the age of 25. By arranging a well coordinated service involving health visitors, teachers and social workers, continuity of care will make certain that the best possible success in each individual is achieved.

It is expected that, under the changes being introduced following the recommendations of the Warnock Committee that the health visitor will play an important role as 'named person' for handicapped children under the age of 5 years (see page 78).

Child abuse (non-accidental injury)

Another area in which cooperation between child health, education and social services departments is essential is in the control of child abuse. This is dealt with in detail in Chapter 13 (see pages 191–196).

5
Health Services for Schoolchildren

The prevention of disease in schoolchildren is the concern of all branches of the health services, but special arrangements are made under the Education Act 1944 to safeguard the health of children at school. Each Health Authority must organize a comprehensive range of integrated health services for children including a *school health service* run in conjunction with the relevant local education authority. Each Health Authority must arrange for the services of a Specialist in Community Medicine (Child Health) who is responsible to the local education authority for providing and organizing the health staff for the school health services. Many doctors are employed within the school health service by the District Health Authority—some being specially trained to deal with handicapped children—and are either employed full-time or part time on a sessional basis and in this respect increasing use is made of general practitioners.

The move of a child to school when aged five years is one of the more important changes in life. He has to leave the comparative peace and security of his own home and mix with dozens of other children in the competitive atmosphere of the classroom and playground. Even for the child with brothers and sisters, the move to school is important, but, for the first or only child, the impact of school represents a very great change.

School life in all children covers the next eleven years and many remain at school until eighteen years of age when they move on to a University.

Preventive medicine for any child of school age is largely connected with school life. In order to help children to get the most benefit from their education, a highly developed preventive medical service has been built up – the *School Health Service* – to ensure that every child's health is safeguarded throughout his school career.

There are two main functions of the school health service:

(a) To make certain that every child is *as fit as possible*. This includes many services designed to diagnose disabilities as early as possible, to allow for correction before they have a lasting effect upon the health of the child. This function also includes the promotion of *positive health*—it is not just sufficient to see that no disease occurs, but there must be a positive programme designed to make every school child as fit as possible.

(b) To assist with the care of various groups of *handicapped children*.

68

Nursery school

The normal child can gain much from attending a nursery school when aged 3–5 years. The value of such schools which the children usually attend for half a day, is in the social contact made. The child gets used to working with others and this is specially useful for the child and makes the entry into primary school easier. The medical care of children in nursery schools is important and is undertaken by the school health service. Special care must be taken with outbreaks of communicable disease as conditions such as dysentery can rapidly spread in nursery schools if not recognized early (see page 113).

Steps taken to ensure every school child is as fit as possible

The present method of medical examination in schools is a combination of *full routine medical examinations* on all children either just before or immediately after entry into school (5 years) combined with *selective medical examinations during school life.* Just before leaving school (15 years) there is another full examination including a fitness test for employment.

Occasionally the initial examination is replaced by a *pre-school initial medical inspection* at 4 years of age. This has the advantage that a dental examination is possible earlier (when conservative dentistry is more effective) and enables any medical defect discovered to be investigated fully and treated before entry to school.

Routine medical inspections

Each school is visited at least once a year by the team carrying out the routine medical inspection—the school doctor, the health visitor and/or school nurse, and a clerk to assist with clerical work. The medical examination takes place at school, if possible in a medical inspection room. Parents are invited to be present and their presence is most important especially with the first medical inspection. It is best to summon parents on a single appointment system so that they are kept waiting as little as possible. About 12 children are examined each morning and afternoon.

A very careful *medical history* is taken from the parent and this is supplemented by records from the child health service and from the general practitioner. These should provide a complete story of the child's progress from infancy with full details of any illness, medical problems, immunizations, as well as a brief record of the health of the parents and family. It is best if the health visitor who dealt with the child when a baby also looks after the school which the child attends. This is not always possible but is usually the case, for the infant's school is normally in the same district as the child's home. To have the same health visitor working with pre-school children and with the infant and junior schools, means that she knows a great deal about the background of each child. Any unusual point in the medical history is noted and problems should be carefully watched.

A full *medical examination* then takes place by the school doctor. All systems are carefully examined, including the special senses. Apart from testing for abnormalities particular attention is paid to posture, nutrition and minor orthopaedic problems such as foot deformities—pes cavus, flat foot. The intelligence of each child is not tested routinely but if the teacher raises any doubt about a child's mental ability a special intelligence test is arranged at once.

Sight testing is carried out routinely on five-year-olds and the Keystone machine which tests visual acuity, colour vision and muscle balance may be used. If any defect is found, a full ophthalmic examination is arranged.

Any child with a squint must be treated immediately. Treatment can be carried out at the nearest eye hospital or special orthoptic treatment can be arranged by the school health service.

The *hearing* of every child should be examined *individually* in the first medical examination when aged five. This can conveniently be carried out by a doctor or health visitor using a sweep test with a portable pure tone audiometer. This is a light portable machine which produces sound of varying volume at frequency ranges from 128 to 8000 cycles per second. Each ear is tested independently—the child being given a small wooden mallet and asked to strike the table each time a sound is heard. Each frequency is tested starting with a loud volume of sound and gradually the volume is reduced until the child can no longer hear anything. This indicates the *threshold of hearing*— the lowest volume of sound at that particular frequency which the child can hear. This test is repeated for each frequency so that a pattern of hearing is established for both ears and at a number of different frequencies. It is important to test at different frequencies as occasionally there is a loss of hearing at one particular part of the sound scale (high-frequency deafness).

Testing the hearing of a five-year-old with this machine in expert hands takes between two and three minutes. About 5 per cent of those tested fail the tests. All who fail should be retested immediately and this usually results in about a third of those who originally failed the test, passing it on the second occasion (they failed the first time not because of hearing loss but because they failed to understand the test). This means about 3 per cent of the original group fail. These children must all be investigated further by an Ear, Nose and Throat Department to establish the cause of their hearing loss. In many cases, the hearing loss is quite small and, without a special test, might never be discovered. It is, however, most important that any hearing loss, even if small, is discovered early, otherwise it is very likely to interfere with the educational progress of the child, because the child will probably not be working to his full potential, although, if intelligent, may still be progressing quite well compared to other children.

All children with a hearing loss are carefully followed up and, where necessary, a hearing aid is prescribed by the hospital department. Those with minimal hearing loss are always put at the front of the class to make certain they have the best opportunity to hear each lesson.

If any illness or disability is discovered in the routine medical examination, the parent is told about it and a note sent to the child's own general practitioner who then arranges for treatment. The school health service is really *a diagnostic service* and not a treatment service, although it is careful to check that the treatment ordered by the doctor is properly carried out by the child. In some cases, the treatment may affect the child's ability to play a full part in the activities of the school—e.g. games. Wherever possible, interference in this way is always kept to a minimum for it is most important that no child should ever think some activity cannot be undertaken unless this is essential. Close liaison must be maintained between the family doctor and school doctor in this respect.

After the school medical examination, the school doctor indicates those children who need to be seen again. Whenever any disability is discovered, arrangements are always made to see the child and parent again in a few weeks after treatment. This succeeding examination will take place at one of the follow-up school clinics held weekly. All children who have been found to have disabilities should be seen on the next routine medical examination which the doctor carries out at that school—this will normally be the following year. A perfectly normal child would not be seen by the doctor following the initial medical inspection at 4 to 5 years until the child is to leave school (15 years).

The exceptions to this would be if a sudden illness developed in the meantime or if the parent or teacher were worried about the health of the child—in this case, the child would be seen either at the next visit of the doctor to school or be referred to the follow-up clinic.

A few examples of how routine medical inspection works are given by:

1 **Normal child.** The child is medically examined at school when aged 5 years and 15 years. In addition the health visitor/school nurse visits the school each term to check on minor illnesses and absentees. A questionnaire is completed by parent and teacher when the child is aged 8 years and 12 years. Selective medical examination is carried out where the answers cause concern.

2 **Child with constant disability.** A child with defective vision, or some chronic disability such as a scoliosis, would be seen when five years old at school, and then on each *annual* routine medical examination carried out by the doctor on the next visit to the school. Also the child may be seen at any time at follow-up clinics.

3 Normal child on entry to school who later develops severe illness. An example would be a child found to be quite normal on entering school at 5 years but who developed rheumatic fever when aged 7. This child would have been medically examined at 5, found normal, and marked to be seen again at 15. However, when rheumatic fever developed at 7, the child would be referred immediately on return to the school doctor and would then be seen regularly as needed and on each subsequent routine medical examination at the school.

This careful 'watching over' process of the health of all schoolchildren should always be carried out in such a way as to help and assist parents, general practitioners and teachers. All children are seen after any recent serious illness, or if the teacher, parent or health visitor/school nurse is concerned because of unsatisfactory progress or difficulty of any kind.

Other functions of the school medical officer

The good school doctor will visit schools in between the more lengthy visits to carry out routine medical inspections and check up other points which are important to the health of the child. These include:

(a) *Helpful advice about the hygiene in the school.* This will include examination of buildings, heating, washing facilities and kitchen premises.

(b) *Investigation of all communicable diseases.* There are always likely to be outbreaks of communicable disease in schools, especially in infant and junior schools. Much time can be saved by prompt and proper investigation. It is not usual today to quarantine large numbers of children, for it is known that this rarely achieves much prevention of disease and always means a great loss of education time. However, bacteriological investigations should be carried out on the close family contacts of certain communicable diseases (such as diphtheria, dysentery, salmonella or enteric infections) and may prevent much unnecessary disease by defining carriers who may spread the disease.

Whenever a case of tuberculosis occurs within a school, complete and careful examination of all contacts (staff and children) must be carried out to make certain that an unsuspected case has not been the cause.

It is best always for all such investigations to be undertaken by the regular school doctor and health visitor for they know so much about the school and its staff and children, and will thus be able to ensure that fullest investigations are undertaken with the minimum interference to school work.

(c) *Health education* should be one of the most important functions of the school health team. *The aim is to promote positive health*—to assist the teaching staff to improve the health of the child as far as possible. This means encouraging certain non-athletic and underdeveloped children to improve their physique in various ways. Every school doctor should take an interest in the games schedules of the school. But it is also important not to neglect that group of children who, for one reason or another (e.g. bad eyesight) never seem able to excel at traditional ball games. Other forms of active recreation should always be encouraged and special activities such as walking, camping, cycling, rock climbing, skiing, fishing, sailing, skating and riding should, wherever possible, be part of the sporting activities of any school. To benefit from such sports is within the compass of any school today, for the Central Council of Physical Recreation runs a multitude of excellent courses in all areas of the country especially designed to introduce the older school child to such activities. Such an introduction may readily play an active part in maintaining the health of the adult later in life.

Special subjects in health education must be tackled such as sex education, care of teeth and education to prevent children starting to smoke. None of these topics is easy to put over successfully and often more can be gained by example. In this respect, the behaviour of all the teaching staff is most important—a campaign to stop children from starting to smoke is unlikely to succeed unless staff are also prepared to help. Attempts must always be made to see that health education comes into ordinary education wherever possible so that it is a continuously active process rather than a sudden strenuous campaign.

(d) *Immunizations* should be encouraged in schoolchildren. Booster doses of diphtheria and poliomyelitis immunization should be given to those who have had prior courses. For children who have never been immunized, primary courses of immunization should be arranged at school. The aim should be to make it as easy as possible for the child to be immunized.

BCG vaccination against tuberculosis should be offered to all school-children aged 12 to 13 years who are then Mantoux negative (see page 105).

Arrangements should be made to immunize all girls against rubella between the ages of 11 and 13.

(e) *The discovery or ascertainment of all groups of handicapped children* is another function of the school doctor.

Routine inspections by health visitors

In addition to the health inspection visit, the health visitor visits each school frequently:

(i) to note which children are absent from school so she can pay a home visit to help and advise;

(ii) to carry out certain screening tests—repeat any hearing tests and test the vision of 7 year old children;

(iii) to carry out regular cleanliness inspections on schoolchildren.

About 2 per cent of all schoolchildren are found to have evidence of infestation with head lice. These infestations are mainly in the form of nits—the eggs of the head louse. Arrangements are then made for the cleansing of the child at a convenient clinic and for subsequent examination to make certain that there has not been a recurrence. It is essential for the health visitor to visit the home, for often members of the family are involved and, in such cases, to treat the schoolchildren only will achieve little. On such visits particular attention must be paid to examine the hair of the older members of the family.

Another disease in which it is important to treat all the family and which occasionally is found in schoolchildren is *scabies*. Modern treatment with benzyl benzoate solution is most efficient and soon controls such infestations, provided *all infected members of the family are treated simultaneously*.

School clinics

School clinics are provided so that schoolchildren can attend follow-up clinics and have minor ailments treated without having to spend much time away from school. Treatment is not really the function of the school health service but there are so many problems connected with getting children's eyes tested for glasses that it has been found most convenient for an eye specialist to hold *an ophthalmic clinic* in a school clinic periodically. The District Health Authority cooperates with the Education Committee in arranging this service.

Occasional special *orthopaedic clinics* are held in school clinics by orthopaedic consultants to treat and follow up the large number of minor orthopaedic problems always found in a school population. Such clinics are of special importance in country areas where attendance at a hospital outpatient department may be difficult.

Preventive dental treatment in schoolchildren

A comprehensive preventive dental service is an important part of the school health service. Unlike the rest of the school health service, the school dental service is both a diagnostic and treatment service.

A visit is paid by the dental surgeon to each school every six months and every child is examined dentally and notes made of all defects. Each child is then called for individual treatment by the dentist in the following weeks. Treatment is free and usually carried out at the dental clinic which normally is attached to the school clinic. In remote country areas dental clinics may be mounted in a mobile caravan so that the treatment centre can be taken and parked at the school. This arrangement allows treatment of every child to be carried out without taking the children away from school for long periods.

Most school dental services have facilities to carry out orthodontic treatment, on children with crowded and misplaced teeth. Effective orthodontic treatment in the school child can prevent many dental problems later. It is, however, most important that orthodontic treatment is started early enough so that the permanent teeth can develop correctly.

There is a shortage of dentists in the school dental service and, to help overcome this, *dental hygienists* work under the personal direction of dentists tackling certain tasks such as the scaling of teeth and doing some fillings.

A recent report of a study of the dental health of children 5–15 years in maintained schools showed that very few children avoid dental decay— seven out of ten of the 5 year old children had evidence of past or present decay. Among teenagers the proportion was more than 95 out of 100. Some evidence of gingivitis was found in half of the children by the age of 17. There was also marked regional variation and this may be connected with either the natural or artificial fluoridation of water supplies.

Care of the handicapped school child

An important subsidiary function of the school health service is to assist in the diagnosis, discovery and special care for all handicapped school children whether the handicap or disability is physical or mental.

The education of children and young people who are handicapped or, to use a more modern phrase, have disabilities or significant difficulties was studied in detail by an expert Committee set up by the Department of Education and Science under the chairmanship of Mary Warnock. This Committee reported in 1978 and, since then, governments have generally accepted many of its recommendations in a White Paper and have introduced the Education Act, 1981 to change the law where this is necessary.

At present, any Local Education Authority (LEA) can legally insist on a medical and other examination of any child whom they have reason to believe requires special education once that child has reached the age of 2 years.

Under the 1981 Education Act, the LEA will continue to be required to determine the special educational provision which needs to be made and to assess the child's needs. However, *parents must be involved in the making of the assessments and may appeal against the decisions*. LEAs will also be empowered, for the first time, *with the consent of parents* to assess these special educational needs of children under 2 years of age and to maintain records and statements about them.

In addition, parents will in future be able to request that the LEA assesses the special needs of their child whether or not statements or records are being maintained for them.

Definition of special educational needs under the 1981 Education Act

The 1981 Education Act accepts the recommendation of the Warnock Committee that the narrow definition of handicapped children (which only includes blind, partially sighted, deaf, partially deaf, delicate, educationally backward, emotionally and behaviourally disturbed, physically handicapped, epileptic, speech defect children) should be extended to include any child who requires some form of special educational provision (including 'remedial' education). This will mean that approximately 16–17% of the school population (one in six) will be involved at any one time (or 20% or one in five at some time during their school life). *Special educational provision* may take the form of special teaching techniques or equipment, a specially modified curriculum or help with social or emotional problems.

Duties of Local Education Authorities (LEAs)

Under the 1981 Education Act all LEAs must assess any child whom the LEA considers has a special educational need. Medical, psychological and educational advice *must* be sought in each assessment and assistance may also be obtained from social services where this is appropriate.

Once any child has been assessed to have a special educational need, the *LEA will be under a legal duty to arrange special educational provision* in accordance with the statement outlining that need. Parents also *must* receive a copy of the statement—indeed much emphasis in the Act is placed on parental involvement and cooperation. Parents *must* also be given the name and address of a person to whom they may apply for information and advice about their child's special educational needs.

The 1981 Education Act requires all LEAs to provide for the needs of children requiring special education and to keep them under review. This should include making arrangements to educate children with special needs with ordinary children (i.e. integration) and parental wishes should be met wherever possible. Where it would be inappropriate for special educational provison to be made at school, LEAs will be able to arrange for it to be made elsewhere.

Recording of handicapped children

A detailed statement will be maintained for each child. This record should contain the results of multi-professional assessment and should carefully define the individual handicaps or disabilities and the child's special needs and difficulties. It should also indicate the special form of education required for the child. The LEA will then have to meet such needs.

Parents will be consulted in the drawing up of the record and it will be a legal requirement, in the future, for the LEA to review, modify and maintain the record. In the event of a disagreement by the parents with the LEA, there will be an appeal to a special appeal committee and a final right of appeal to the Secretary of State.

Principles applying to meeting special educational needs

Certain basic principles apply to the education of children with special needs:

1 every effort should be made to discover the extent of the disability and *special needs of the child as early as possible*. In some instances, such as congenital deafness, this will be within the first year of life;
2 special *education and care should be started early* and *continued well after the normal school leaving age*;
3 the aim should be to make each child as independent as possible;
4 each child should be dealt with individually and improvisation is always helpful;
5 the best solution is usually that which is as near normal as possible. All forms of integration into the ordinary school system are therefore very useful;
6 the after-care of children with disabilities or significant difficulties when they leave school is most important. Wherever possible, special vocational training and/or work preparation should be arranged.

To encourage early discovery and identification of special educational needs, all DHAs, under the Education Act 1981, have a legal duty to inform parents and the LEA where they form the opinion that a child under the age of 5 has, or is likely to have, special educational needs. The DHA must also afford the parents an opportunity to discuss their opinion *before* bringing the child to the attention of the LEA.

There are many ways in which a handicapped child can be educated: (a) in an ordinary school; (b) in a special class in an ordinary school; (c) in a day special school; (d) in a residential special school; (e) at home with a peripatetic teacher or in a combination of these.

Discovery of disabilities and disclosure to parents

The importance of early discovery of any disability in a child has already been stressed. Depending on the nature of the handicap or problem, it may be discovered shortly after birth by the parents, doctors, health visitor or during the first few years or not even until the child attends a day nursery, nursery school or primary school. In all instances, it is essential that a full explanation is given in a sensitive way to the parents. Many may find it difficult to grasp the full meaning and significance, especially in the case of a serious disability and such parents *will need constant support* and will require *information, advice and practical help*. It is best if parents have nominated one individual professional to act as a 'Named Person' who can introduce the parents to the right services, explain any problems and generally act as a guide and counsellor. For any child of pre-school age, the *health visitor* will normally act in this capacity, although in exceptional cases (e.g. a deaf child) another professional (e.g. peripatetic teacher) may act as Named Person. For children with special needs at school, the head teacher should undertake this role. Parents should be encouraged to discuss their doubts and fears openly for concealment only adds to their problems.

Assessment of special educational needs

The assessment of a child with a disability or significant difficulty should be undertaken in the following way:

1   *Parents should always be involved* for no estimation of a child's needs can be complete without the fullest help from parents. The aim should be to treat parents as partners *and parents must be kept fully informed of all expert investigation;*
2   *Multi-professional assessment should always be undertaken.* This will include expert medical examination by hospital paediatricians as well as assessment by health visitors, educational psychologists, teachers, social work staff and day nursery matrons, where appropriate. Assessment should aim at discovering how the child learns and responds over a period of time;
3   There must be full *investigations of any aspect of the child's perform-ance which is causing concern;*
4   The family and home circumstances should always be taken into account.

The 1981 Education Act includes a clause which enables parents to request that the needs of their children be assessed, whether or not statements (records) are being maintained for them.

Range of special education provided

The special educational needs of children are extremely complex and varied. It may be possible for even the seriously disabled to be educated in ordinary schools provided special ramps are available to accommodate wheelchairs, special teaching equipment is available and transport is provided to enable the child to get to school.

For most children with severe disabilities and for those who have already attended a primary school but made little progress, attendance at a special school may be needed at least for an initial period. Special schools are provided directly by LEAs and voluntary bodies and, under the 1981 Education Act, the Secretary of State is empowered to make regulations in respect of the approval of special schools and independent schools.

In general, special schools are needed for three groups:

1 children with very severe or complex disabilities. This group includes a wide range of conditions including complete blindness or deafness, severe congenital disabilities such as spina bifida and the worst cerebral palsies, and progressive diseases such as Duchenne muscular dystrophy;
2 children with severe emotional or behavioural disorders whose behaviour is extreme and unpredictable. Such children were formerly called 'maladjusted' but this is a term no longer in general use;
3 children who for various reasons have done badly in ordinary school and who need the more intimate atmosphere of smaller teaching groups.

Integration

Wherever possible, children with special educational needs should be educated in ordinary schools (integration). There are three forms of integration:

1 *Locational*—where a special school unit is sited within the same grounds as an ordinary school, but is still run as a separate school. This is a first step in integration and is helpful in reducing isolation and stigma felt by parents and children who attend a 'special school'. It also enables seriously disabled children to attend the 'same school' as their brothers and sisters. It also helps the children in ordinary schools to understand better the needs and problems of handicapped children;
2 *Social integration* is a further step and here the children play, eat and mix with the children from the adjacent ordinary school and may even share some of their out-of-classroom activities. Classroom teaching, however, remains separate;
3 *Functional integration* achieves all the above mixing but, in addition, the disabled children share most of their classes with ordinary children. Such an arrangement still allows some specialized teaching but enables the handicapped children to gain access to a wider range of teaching than is usually possible in a special school. It also enables

the potential of most disabled children to be better reached.

For severely disabled children who have to spend most of their school life in a special school, it is important for them to experience some degree of social and functional integration during the last two to three years at school. This is the best way to avoid overprotection of such children which, to some degree, is inevitable for any child attending a small special school.

Special problems of the disabled child in the transitional period from school into adult life

All children with disabilities or significant difficulties meet special problems on leaving school. They are likely to find more difficulty in getting a job or in being accepted for higher education. Careful preparation is therefore important and re-assessment should always take place during the last two or three years at school. As well as the usual professionals, careers guidance officers, Disablement Resettlement Officers and special social workers from the social services department should be involved.

Special linked courses whereby children may spend part of their time in a nearby college of further education and 'work preparation' schemes can be of considerable value. For disabled young persons over school leaving age, there are also Employment Rehabilitation Centres run by the Employment Service Division of the Manpower Services Commission. There are also a number of specialized residential assessment courses at special units such as the Queen Elizabeth's Foundation at Banstead Place. *Special Careers Officers* are employed by most LEAs to give special help to disabled school leavers.

Young persons who are mentally handicapped and have been attending special schools will usually transfer to local Adult Training Centres run by social services departments (see page 238) and hopefully later to sheltered workshops.

Importance of further education

Many disabled young persons will find it difficult to find work unless they can become qualified in some way. Therefore, they should, wherever possible, be encouraged to attend a college of further education or some form of higher education (polytechnic or university).

At Coventry, the LEA runs a very modern residential further education college (Hereward College). There are also a number of voluntary bodies who run excellent residential training colleges.

Special groups of children with disabilities or significant difficulties

Although handicapped children are no longer categorized, those with certain types of disabilities still require specialized help and brief notes are given below describing these.

Children who are blind or partially sighted

Blind children have no useful sight and must be educated by non-visual methods. Education in nearly all cases takes place in a residential school except in the largest cities. Blind children often start their training at the age of two years in the Sunshine Homes run by the Royal National Institute for the Blind.

Partially sighted children have very poor eyesight but, with special assistance, they can be taught using visual methods. Classes must be very small, not more than ten in a class, and special equipment is needed. In most instances, partially sighted children can be taught in special day schools or special classes within day schools.

Children who are deaf or partially deaf

Deaf children have no useful hearing and cannot be taught by auditory methods. It is essential that their training and education should start very young (as soon as diagnosed) and it is very specialized. By remarkable methods which have translated the teaching of sounds into visual tuition, it has been possible to teach speech to totally deaf children who have never heard human speech. In the absence of such teaching, the totally deaf child will also be dumb, as speaking is learnt by the child copying what he hears. Most deaf children are educated in special residential schools.

Partially deaf children can be educated in small classes using auditory methods provided special hearing aids are available. Such tuition usually takes place in special day schools but may be carried out in residential schools.

Delicate children

This group is a large mixed group containing many medical and surgical conditions which interfere with a child's education. Chest diseases (such as asthma, bronchiectasis and tuberculosis), heart conditions (rheumatic heart or congenital heart disease), blood diseases, diabetes and alimentary diseases make up this group, which includes any rare disease of childhood which makes a child's education difficult.

Many of these children need at first to be admitted to a residential school to allow their medical and educational condition to be fully assessed. In many instances, the child's education will have been very badly interrupted by repeated illnesses and the child becomes very backward in his education. Many parents of such children worry so much about the child's health that they overprotect the child.

Having assessed the child in a residential school and having introduced some degree of stability into his education, it is often possible later to return the child to a special day school.

In the case of a child undergoing a series of serious operations—such as a bronchiectatic child—the regime at a residential school will often build him up and help his treatment as well as maintaining, as far as possible, continuity with his education.

Children with intellectual impairment

The degree of intellectual impairment in children can vary from those who have difficulties in learning and keeping up with their peers at school to those who need long term specialist education in order to accomplish even the most basic of everyday personal skills. Children in this last group are usually said to be 'mentally handicapped'.

Many children who are handicapped in these ways exhibit more behaviour difficulties than normal children. Their rate of juvenile delinquency is always higher and a continuing problem for the school health and social services. Girls tend to reach sexual maturity quite early and may be in moral danger, being more easily led astray. It is important therefore that this is anticipated and fully discussed with the parents or guardian to reduce such a risk. Surveys of adolescent unmarried mothers have tended to show that a greater proportion of these children have some form of intellectual impairment.

Until recently children with intellectual handicap were classified rather rigidly as 'educationally subnormal (moderate)—ESN(M)', and 'educationally subnormal (severe)—ESN(S)' (e.g. mental handicap). These terms should not be used in future. It is now recognised that many children can achieve far more if, from the outset, all their qualities, such as their social adjustment, emotional and behavioural patterns are taken into consideration when deciding what type of educational opportunities or help may be open to them. More severe intellectual handicap or 'mental handicap' is also covered in Chapter 15. It should be noted that whilst 'intellectual handicap' or 'impairment' are frequently used in preference to 'mental handicap', they should not be confused with 'mental impairment' as defined in the Mental Health Act 1983, see page 229.

Intelligence Tests

Although it should not be isolated from other aspects of a person's character and behavioural pattern, the intelligence test is a means of estimating the mental age of a child or adult. It consists of a series of tests, questions and exercises designed to demonstrate knowledge gained and reasoning power.

The *Intelligence Quotient* $= \dfrac{\text{Mental Age}}{\text{Real Age}} \times 100$.

Examples

A child aged 10 years who has a mental age of 12 years would have an intelligence quotient (IQ) of 120.

$$\text{IQ} = \frac{\text{Mental Age}}{\text{Real Age}} \times 100 = \frac{12}{10} \times 100 = 120.$$

A child aged 10 years who has a mental age of 10 years would have an intelligence quotient of 100.

$$\text{IQ} = \frac{\text{Mental Age}}{\text{Real Age}} \times 100 = \frac{10}{10} \times 100 = 100.$$

A child aged 10 years who has a mental age of 8 years would have an intelligence quotient of 80.

$$\text{IQ} = \frac{\text{Mental Age}}{\text{Real Age}} \times 100 = 80.$$

It will thus be seen that a perfectly normal average child would have an Intelligence quotient of 100. Above average intelligence gives an intelligence quotient over 100 and below average intelligence an intelligence quotient below 100.

Value of the intelligence quotient. Intelligence quotients vary roughly as follows:

120–125 +	University entrant
115 +	Bright school child
90–115 +	Average school child
80–90	Retarded school child
55–79 ⎫	Intellectual impairment/mental handicap of
Under 50–55 ⎭	varying degree

It is, however, important to realize that *these levels are guides only* and that exceptions occur in this grouping.

In grading a backward child, it is necessary to carry out probably two or more intelligence tests and also to try the child out with a highly experienced teacher before the final decision is made. A very careful search must always be made for any signs of an accompanying physical deformity, such as deafness, which could be responsible for the low result.

Intellectually handicapped children may need to be educated in either a residential or special day school where the curriculum contains a greater proportion of practical teaching, and where the pace of the teaching is slower than at a normal school.

A child who does well in special school may later be able to move back to an ordinary school.

Children with severe emotional or behavioural disorders

A child in this group is one who is a 'problem child' showing many behaviour difficulties. Because of this, he may become retarded educationally, although his intelligence may be normal.

There are many causes of this problem. Some of these children show emotional instability and even a psychological disorder, but many just reflect unstable home conditions including marital difficulties, divorce or separation of parents.

Complete careful diagnosis of the problem is essential. This is rarely a simple procedure. Often repeated visits of the child and his parents to the *Child Guidance Clinic*, where a psychiatrist and psychiatric social worker are in attendance, will be necessary before the complete causative factors are unravelled. It is usual for the social worker attached to the child guidance clinic to be a member of the Social Services Department so that there is maximium coordination between the social work undertaken in the child guidance clinics and the community social services.

These children are best educated in ordinary schools for they gain from contact with normal children although if their home is very unsatisfactory they may have to be in residential (boarding) school. Any psychological disorders in the children must be treated appropriately. It will, however, be necessary to attempt to improve the home conditions. Because it is often hard or impossible to improve conditions in a divided home, treatment is often difficult and calls for much patience. Relapses in behaviour occur and delinquency may complicate the picture. Continued encouragement and understanding by teaching and medical staff will sometimes eventually succeed.

Failure in such children may have serious consequences later for they may drift into criminal behaviour and may even become chronic criminals. There is no doubt that much crime could be prevented by more concentrated medico-social work upon school-children who exhibit extreme forms of behaviour.

Children who are physically handicapped

This group contains the very severely handicapped children. Many have serious handicaps, often with paralysis, and include children handicapped by such diseases as poliomyelitis, muscular dystrophies and other serious orthopaedic conditions. Many such children have not attended normal schools since their illness commenced. It is usual to educate such children in special residential or day schools in which the classes are very small so that each crippled child can receive much personal attention.

In those diseases which are not progressive, it is important towards the end of the child's education to do everything possible to make him as independent as possible. In this respect, it is always wise to try and arrange for the child to spend his last year of school life at an ordinary school even if this can only be achieved by much improvisation—such as organising special transport. If the child can learn such independence, he is far more likely to succeed in finding and holding a job on leaving school.

Children with epilepsy

The majority of children with epilepsy can be educated in an ordinary school provided that:

(a) the fits do not occur very often;
(b) there is no marked behaviour difficulty—i.e., the emotional stability of the child is reasonably normal;
(c) there is a good liaison between the school doctor and teacher who realizes that no other child in the class will come to any harm from witnessing the occasional epileptic fit.

In the case of very frequent major fits or of marked emotional instability, it is wise to arrange for the child to be admitted at once to a special residential school for epileptic children for assessment and treatment. Such a school may be run in conjunction with an epileptic colony and its medical and teaching staff will have great experience of such problems. After assessment and correct treatment, in a proportion of cases, it will be possible for the child to return to an ordinary school.

It is, however, stressed that only a small proportion of children with epilepsy ever need to go to such a school, for most can be educated at an ordinary school quite satisfactorily.

Children with speech defects

Any defect of speech in a school child can be serious unless corrected. Such children may quickly develop emotional difficulties from the frustration of being unable to make themselves readily understood. This in turn will tend to aggravate their speech defect.

A most careful physical examination is needed to exclude a physical cause (defective hearing or deformities of palate) and then regular speech therapy must be started. Speech therapists are on the staff of each school health service to carry out this treatment by relaxation training and speech training.

It is most important that the child with a speech defect stays in a normal school with normal children. Special schools are, therefore, not needed.

Children with dyslexia

Dyslexia is an interesting condition in which there is a specific language difficulty which shows itself in a series of ways affecting spelling, reading and other language skills. There is always a marked discrepancy between the mental potential of the child (which is often normal) and his educational level despite conventional classroom instruction. The incidence of dyslexia is as high as 3 per cent although many minor cases are missed. In many instances the condition is not recognised until very late with consequent serious loss of learning potential. In many such cases these children may later become language-disabled adults.

The cause of dyslexia is not fully understood but most agree that it is caused by a lesion in the central nervous system which has been present either from birth or shortly afterwards. Many children suffering from dyslexia do well if the condition is recognized early, they attend nursery schools and later receive *individual teaching* or teaching in very small groups in which it is possible to mould a teaching programme to an individual child.

6
Prevention of Disease by Immunization

In many communicable diseases, an attack of the disease is followed by a varying period of immunity from further attacks. Not all communicable diseases are followed by an immunity (for example, the common cold is followed by only a very transient immunity) but in many, the length of immunity is substantial, lasting years or even a lifetime. Whenever a person develops an immunity in this way, the body manufactures special disease resistant bodies called *antibodies*.

It is possible to copy this mechanism artificially by introducing into the human body modified bacteria, viruses or their products so that the individual does not suffer from the disease but does develop antibodies and, therefore, does develop an immunity to a natural attack.

Artificial immunization and vaccination relies on this principle. Immunity can be either *active* or *passive*.

In **active immunity** a special product of the bacteria or virus (*antigen*) is introduced into the body, often by injection, but occasionally by mouth, which stimulates the human body to manufacture its own protective antibodies. Immunity produced in this way is always more satisfactory as it lasts a long time. *Its only drawback is that it often takes two to three months for the human body to build up such immunity.*

Passive immunity is used when an animal, such as an ox, has first been actively immunized and has itself manufactured antibodies, which are then used to protect man. The great value of this method is that it gives immediate immunity, but this is very transient and rarely lasts longer than about four to six weeks. It is, however, very useful either to treat a patient suffering from the disease, such as diphtheria antitoxin, or to give a temporary immunity to a person who has been in close contact with the disease and who may be incubating it. A disadvantage is that the patient may easily be sensitized to the protein of the animal and suffer from serum sickness.

A more satisfactory passive immunity is obtained by using *immunoglobulin*, the active constituent of human blood which contains the antibodies.

In preventive medicine, greater use is made of active immunization than passive immunization.

Active immunization

The dangers of communicable disease arise in two main ways:

(i) by a direct invasion process of a certain part of the body. Examples include inflammation of lung in whooping cough, of the small intestine in typhoid or of part of the central nervous system in encephalitis.

(ii) by the bacteria producing a very powerful poison (toxin) usually as it grows in the body. Examples include diphtheria, tetanus or toxin food poisoning.

The first group of diseases is usually prevented by using an antigen which consists of either the dead bacteria or viruses concerned (typhoid prevented by Typhoid Paratyphoid A & B Vaccine (TAB), or whooping cough by whooping cough vaccine), or else by a modified or changed live bacteria such as Bacillus Calmette-Guérin (BCG) in tuberculosis, or live virus as in Sabin vaccine in poliomyelitis. In the latter two cases, the live bacteria or virus has been changed (undergone a mutation) which results in the modified bacteria or virus being unable to produce the real disease in the human, but it can still produce a modified reaction which then will be followed by an immunity.

Some quite startling successes have been achieved by immunization. Diphtheria is probably the best example. In the ten years before immunization started in 1943, approximately 50 000 cases occurred each year. This meant that about one person in ten might ordinarily have been expected to suffer from diphtheria at some time during his life. After immunization was introduced, the incidence fell rapidly. This improvement has continued and in 1980 two cases were traced. Immunization has virtually eradicated the disease.

Although other diseases have not diminished so dramatically, there has been a similar improvement in poliomyelitis which has now become very rare.

It is important to realize that people inherit different amounts of natural immunity. A few fortunate people have a remarkable natural immunity while many others have little or none. When all people are immunized their natural immunity is added to very considerably. This means that, after immunization, there will still be considerable variation in the amount of immunity in any group which has just been immunized. Over a period of years, protection will gradually wear off. Obviously the person who had very little natural immunity will have his acquired immunity lowered more quickly in this way, to a level where an attack of the disease will not be averted.

This is the reason why, after immunization, it is never possible to guarantee complete protection in everyone. Most diseases are usually avoided in 90 per cent of people by immunization, and even in those who do develop an attack after immunization, it is usually a much milder attack.

Active immunization schedule for a child

Age	Immunization
3–6 months	Triple immunization (diphtheria, whooping cough and tetanus) plus oral poliomyelitis (1)
5–8 months	Triple immunization (diphtheria, whooping cough and tetanus) plus oral poliomyelitis (2)
12 months	Triple immunization (diphtheria, whooping cough and tetanus) plus oral poliomyelitis (3)
14 to 18 months	Measles
5 years	Booster: Diphtheria, tetanus and poliomyelitis (oral or inactivated vaccine)
11–13 years	(girls only) Rubella (german measles)
11–13 years	BCG vaccine (to protect against tuberculosis)
15 years	Booster: Tetanus and poliomyelitis (oral or inactivated vaccine)

Triple immunization against diphtheria, whooping cough and tetanus

These immunizations are combined for convenience. They are given first to the young baby at six months because of the importance of avoiding whooping cough early in life when it can be a dangerous disease. However, if immunizations are carried out before this age, the antibody response (and therefore effectiveness) is slight.

The diphtheria and tetanus portions of this immunization are toxoids protecting against the powerful toxins in both diseases. It is impracticable to inject toxin for it has many dangers. If, however, formalin is added to toxin, its chemical composition is changed and the resultant toxoid is quite harmless, but fortunately it will act as an efficient antigen and produce a good immunity.

The whooping cough portion of the immunization is a true vaccine—it is a mixture of killed whooping cough bacteria. Injection of such vaccine leads to a good immunity for four to five years. This means that immunization will postpone the danger of an attack of whooping cough until after the age of five years, so avoiding the dangerous attacks which occur in very young children.

Whooping cough vaccine should not be given to children with a personal or family history of convulsions, cerebral irritation in the neonatal period, epilepsy or any other disorder of the central nervous system.

The diphtheria immunization requires a booster dose periodically and this is given when the child is aged 5 years and 15 years.

Tetanus immunization is boosted by inoculations at 5 and 15 years and afterwards when injury occurs and there is therefore a danger of developing tetanus.

It is most important to realize that all three doses of the primary immunization at 6 months, 8 months and 12 months must be given to ensure complete protection. The first of these injections is followed immediately by hardly any protection—the first dose seems to prepare the body's mechanism for producing antibodies. The second dose is followed immediately by a fair protection but it is the third dose which produces the most lasting protection. For this reason, mothers must make certain that their children have all three doses. A system of computerization of all immunization records helps to remind parents of the need for further immunizations in their children.

Poliomyelitis

This disease was a serious threat until widespread immunization was introduced in the early 1960s. Since then only occasional cases have been reported in the United Kingdom. The continued absence of this disease in any epidemic form is due to the success of poliomyelitis vaccination.

Originally dead inactivated (Salk) vaccine was used but in 1962 this was superseded by Sabin oral vaccine which has the following advantages:

1   it is easier to administer—by mouth rather than injection;
2   it produces an immunity not only to a clinical attack of poliomyelitis, but also to a carrier state in the intestine;
3   it can be given to close contacts to reduce the danger of an epidemic;
4   it is free from dangers of allergic reactions.

There are three types of poliomyelitis virus—type I, II and III—and all three must be included in any vaccine. The mechanism of protection in the oral vaccine is that after each dose the small intestine is seeded with one of the particular types of virus which then grows rapidly and colonizes the intestine. This is followed by a marked immunity to that type of virus.

Once the intestine has been seeded by virus of a particular type, it cannot be colonized again with the same type, so the second dose leads to colonization of one of the other types and the third dose with colonization and protection against all three types.

It is essential that three doses are given to ensure complete protection. The vaccine is given conveniently on a lump of sugar (three drops) or in a sugar solution. Care should be taken to store it in a refrigerator to maintain its potency.

Tuberculosis

Immunization against tuberculosis is undertaken using a live vaccine of the Bacillus Calmette-Guérin (BCG) type. This strain of bacteria is named after the two Frenchmen who first developed it at the beginning of the century. It is a *modified or attenuated strain* of tubercle bacillus which has lost its power to cause the disease in man but can produce a small trivial skin lesion after injection. This local skin infection later leads to an immunity against tuberculosis.

BCG immunization is only used on people who have no skin sensitivity to tuberculin as shown by the tuberculin test. Four main groups of people are immunized against tuberculosis:

1 Close contacts (e.g., other members of the family) of a case of tuberculosis. This group includes the new-born baby born to parents, either of whom has had tuberculosis in the past.
2 Schoolchildren aged 10–13 years, who are tuberculin negative. This represents approximately 8 per cent of schoolchildren. With the parent's consent, all children aged 12 years are given a skin test at school. Those who are tuberculin negative are then vaccinated with BCG.
3 People who in their occupation are liable to run a greater risk of infection from the disease—examples include nurses and doctors in training. It is usual to give a tuberculin test to all new nursing and medical students and to give BCG vaccination to any who are negative. With the increase of routine BCG vaccination to schoolchildren aged 12 years, fewer and fewer nursing and medical students need BCG vaccination on entry.
4 Children of certain immigrants in whose communities there is a high incidence of tuberculosis (especially those from Pakistan, Bangladesh, India and Africa).

After vaccination with BCG, a small skin lesion develops which may suppurate for some weeks and may not clear up until a few months after vaccination. This is quite normal and all that is required is a dry dressing to cover the lesion. Sometimes BCG vaccination is followed by an axillary adenitis. This is rare and usually clears up without complications.

Measles

Immunization against measles is carried out using live vaccines (Scharz strain) given by a single injection at the age of 1 year or shortly afterwards. This usually produces a satisfactory immunity. No child suffering from active tuberculosis or with an allergic history should be immunized against measles.

Rubella (german measles)

Vaccination against rubella should be given to girls aged 11–13 years to avoid any danger later of infection during early pregnancy. A single dose of freeze-dried live attenuated virus of the Cendehill strain is used.

Routine vaccination of adult women is *not* recommended as it is uncertain whether the strain of virus can reach or harm the foetus. If vaccination is requested, a screening serological test should first be carried out by the Public Health Laboratory Service and vaccination should only be offered to those who are seronegative (approx. 10 per cent). *It is most important that a woman is not pregnant at the time of vaccination and does not become pregnant for at least two months after immunization.*

Rabies

Considerable concern is being felt at the present time in the United Kingdom because rabies is widespread on the continent. Although it is hoped to limit this danger by the Rabies Act 1974, it is important for nurses to know that, although rabies can be prevented by *early* active immunization immediately after contact with a rabid animal, the course of injections is long and painful.

Human diploid cell vaccine should be used and the course consists of 14 daily injections into the abdominal wall with a booster dose 10 days later and a final booster 20 days after that.

For people at special risk (handling animals that may be rabid) two immunizations of duck embryo vaccine are given 4–6 weeks apart. Booster doses are given six months later and then every three years.

Anthrax

Immunization against anthrax has now been introduced for all workers at risk. Three doses of killed vaccine is used with 2nd and 3rd injections after 6 and then 20 weeks. A single booster injection is given annually.

Consent to immunizations

As legally an injection is an assault on the person, it is necessary to obtain the written consent from a parent or guardian before immunizing any child or young person under the age of 16 years. Consent is not required in adults.

With oral immunization, consent is not so important although in the case of children it is usual to obtain the consent of the parent. This can conveniently be obtained by circulating letters from school. Recently there has been a move to obtain consent to cover all immunizations necessary for a child, and this practice is likely to spread as it is a much simpler arrangement.

Immunization for people travelling outside this country

There are three diseases for which immunizations are given as protection:

1 Typhoid fever
2 Yellow fever
3 Cholera

1 Typhoid fever. Typhoid and paratyphoid fevers can be prevented by giving a course of Typhoid Paratyphoid ABC vaccine (TAB) which is a suspension of killed bacteria.

Two doses are given at not less than ten day intervals but not more than two months. Booster doses should be given every two years.

TAB immunization should be given to all persons who are going to travel in countries in which primitive water supplies are used. These include all tropical countries, and Italy, Spain, N. Africa and Greece. It is also a wise precaution if camping in Europe.

It is usual to suffer from a mild reaction after TAB inoculations – the patient complains of headache and has a slight pyrexia for a few hours.

2 Yellow fever. Yellow fever is a serious tropical virus disease which is limited to a narrow band of country in mid-Africa and central South America. An effective immunization is given by injection of a live attenuated virus. Very stringent storage conditions are essential for this vaccine which is freeze dried. For this reason, special centres have been set up in this country to give yellow fever vaccination and it can only be given at such centres.

Immunization is only necessary for persons visiting those parts of Africa or South America where the disease occurs. For all such travellers, immunization against yellow fever is compulsory.

3 Cholera. Immunization against cholera is only necessary for travellers who are visiting certain parts of the Indian subcontinent or other far eastern countries in which cholera occurs.

The immunization is by means of a vaccine (a suspension of killed cholera bacteria) and consists of two inoculations with at least two weeks in-between each dose. Moderately severe reactions may follow this inoculation.

Vaccination has proved relatively ineffective against the El Tor strain.

Passive immunization

Reference has already been made to the use of tetanus antitoxin which can be used to prevent attacks of those diseases in a person who has not been immunized but who is at risk. In diphtheria only, antitoxin is a valuable therapeutic agent in the early stages of the disease.

A very useful form of passive immunization is an extract from human blood immunoglobulin which contains the antibodies of infectious diseases. Immunoglobulin, to be of any value in active immunization, must have been separated from the blood of a person who has suffered from the disease.

Examples of the use of immunoglobulin to prevent disease include:

Rubella (german measles)

This is a minor communicable disease and the only reason for ever wishing to prevent an attack is in the case of a woman who is in the early stage of pregnancy. This is because an attack of rubella during the first three months of pregnancy will often result in either a miscarriage or the birth of a congenitally malformed child.

For this reason, if any woman in the first three months of pregnancy is known to have been in contact with a case of rubella and has never suffered from the disease, or has not previously been actively immunized against rubella (see page 91) she should at once be given 2.0 g of immunoglobulin. This will protect her for about six to eight weeks, which is long enough to avoid the danger of any birth complication.

There is only a danger of congenital malformations in the child from an attack of german measles in the first three/four months of pregnancy. An attack later in pregnancy is harmless and, therefore, there is no need to immunize a woman contact then.

Measles

Immunoglobulin is occasionally used to prevent an infant or young child (who has not previously been immunized actively against the disease) catching measles because of the special dangers in individual cases, especially when measles occurs within a paediatric ward which contains a number of unprotected ill children. The sudden complication of an attack of measles would be undesirable for it might prove dangerous in an already ill and debilitated child. To prevent this, the other children within the ward are immunized with immunoglobulin (collected from people who have suffered from measles) and this immediately gives them an immunity for about six weeks. The usual dose in a child under two years is 0.4 g and 0.75 g in older children. In such circumstances, this is a valuable preventive health measure.

Infective hepatitis

It is possible to protect a small vulnerable population (such as those attending a day centre for physically or mentally handicapped persons) against an epidemic of infective hepatitis by using immunoglobulin. In a recent outbreak, success was achieved by actively immunizing those at the centre and newly admitted entrants during the 50 days following the outbreak. The dosage used was 250 mg for babies under the age of one year, 500 mg for infants aged 1 to 2 years, and 750 mg for children aged 3 years and over.

Rabies

Human antirabies immunoglobulin can be used in the post-exposure treatment of persons who are manifestly sensitive to equine antiserum as shown by a skin test. Eventually it is planned to use human antirabies immunoglobulin exclusively.

Chickenpox

Children with leukaemia who are under active treatment with steroids and cytotoxic drugs are very vulnerable and should be given immunoglobulin if exposed to chickenpox infection.

Arrangements for giving immunizations

Immunizations for children can be given:

(a) by the family general practitioner at his own surgery;
(b) at district health authority child health clinics when mothers attend with babies.

There is no special advantage in the immunization being undertaken at child health centres and general practitioners often arrange a special weekly time at their surgeries for immunizations, so that mothers may then bring their children there for immunization without having to mix with ill persons attending ordinary surgery sessions. The doctors have to give immunizations free as part of their service but are paid a small fee for the record card of each completed immunization or vaccination.

7
Prevention of Communicable Diseases

Methods of prevention have been more highly developed in those diseases which are communicable or infectious (which can be passed from person to person or from animal to person) than in other illnesses.

More than two generations ago, it was felt that isolation was likely to be the most valuable single factor, and strict isolation of the patient and his contacts (quarantine) was widely practised. With more and more information as to the exact methods by which these diseases spread, it was realized that isolation is of little value in many communicable diseases.

The role of the infectious disease hospital has completely changed in the last forty years. When isolation was considered to be essential, large infectious disease hospitals were built, often in out-of-the-way districts, so that the isolation of the patients treated in them could be more complete. Today the main reason for arranging admission to such hospitals or wards is not isolation, but because the patient needs hospital treatment as he cannot obtain adequate treatment at home. This is usually because:

(a) treatment of the disease requires specialized techniques—such as severe cases of food poisoning, typhoid fever, anthrax, diphtheria or special complications of measles, whooping cough, scarlet fever or tuberculosis.

(b) the home and social conditions are inadequate to look after the case. Any communicable disease may have to be treated in hospital if the home conditions are unsuitable.

In the case of viral haemorrhagic diseases, complete isolation in a specially designated hospital unit is essential.

Dangers of treating communicable diseases in ordinary wards

It is very undesirable to treat any case of communicable disease in an ordinary ward or even in a side ward of an ordinary ward in a general hospital. Treatment of the patient can quite easily be carried out in an ordinary ward but the danger is that the infection is likely to spread to other patients (cross infection).

Because of this difficulty, modern hospital practice is to have small single bedded disease units—say two wards each containing twelve single rooms attached to a large central hospital. It is also very helpful to have such units attached to a large paediatric hospital. Then any sudden infection in a patient already in the hospital can be treated in the communicable disease unit without interrupting the treatment of the main condition, as the same consultant paediatrician can continue to look after the patient.

Methods of spread of communicable disease

Before the methods of prevention for individual diseases can be discussed, it is necessary to study generally the methods of spread of communicable disease in the United Kingdom.

There are three main groups:

1 **Airborne or droplet infection**
Streptococcal infections—scarlet fever, erysipelas, puerperal fever, tonsillitis
Staphylococcal infections—pemphigus neonatorum
Pneumococcal infections—pneumonia
Diphtheria
Meningitis
Tuberculosis
Common childhood infectious diseases—measles, whooping cough, mumps, rubella.

2 **Faecalborne**—*gastro-intestinal infections*
Typhoid and paratyphoid fever
Food poisoning
Dysentery
Infantile gastro-enteritis
Poliomyelitis
Infective hepatitis

3 **Direct spread by contact**
(a) From animals—*anthrax*
From milk—*undulant fever—brucellosis*
From rats—*leptospirosis*
From rabid dogs and other infected animals—*rabies*
(b) From humans—*sexually transmitted disease—syphilis* and *gonorrhoea*

As will have been seen from the previous chapter (Chapter 6) immunization plays an important rôle in preventing many airborne and faecalborne diseases.

Epidemiological investigation is the second method by which communicable diseases are prevented and their spread controlled. *Epidemiology* is the study of all factors which affect disease—the cause of the illness and all the conditions associated with its incidence. A full investigation is undertaken in all cases so that, as far as possible, the exact method of spread of the disease in the patient can be traced. If this is possible, it will often prevent further cases, for some person may be infectious without showing any symptoms at all—he may be a *carrier*.

Before any investigation can be started, it is, of course, essential to know where all cases have occurred. For this reason, the majority of communicable diseases are compulsorily *notifiable*—they must be reported immediately on diagnosis to the District Medical Officer. A small fee is paid to the doctor for each notification.

Sexually transmitted diseases have never been made notifiable in this country because it is feared that, if they were made so, it would result in concealment of infections and inadequate treatment. Certainly those countries which have introduced notification have a higher level of sexually transmitted disease than the United Kingdom.

The complete list of notifiable diseases is:

Acute meningitis	Ophthalmia neonatorum
Anthrax	Plague
Cholera	Poliomyelitis (acute)
Diphtheria	Rabies
Dysentery (amoebic or bacillary)	Relapsing fever
Encephalitis (acute)	Scarlet fever
Food poisoning	Tetanus
Infective jaundice	Tuberculosis
Lassa fever	Typhoid or paratyphoid
Leprosy	Typhus
Leptospirosis	Viral haemorrhagic fever
Malaria	Whooping cough
Marburg disease	Yellow fever
Measles	

The following communicable diseases are NOT notifiable:

Common cold	Influenza
Chickenpox	Pneumonia
Rubella (german measles)	Sexually transmitted
Mumps	diseases

Method of investigation

A very careful *history* should always be taken from the patient and his close contacts. Any link between the patient and other cases of the disease is carefully investigated. If the disease is one not normally present in this country, such as malaria or typhoid, any link with someone who has recently travelled abroad is followed up. In a gastro-intestinal infection such as food poisoning or typhoid, which is usually the result of a food contamination, a complete history is taken of the food eaten.

In any communicable disease, there is a latent period between infection and the first symptoms and signs of the disease, called *the incubation period*. Thus a person infected with typhoid will show no abnormal signs until fourteen days later when the early symptoms of illness first appear.

A knowledge of the likely incubation period is most important for it allows the questioning in collecting the history to be concentrated where it is most likely to be helpful—at the start of the incubation period (when the patient became infected). When the first symptoms of typhoid appear it is necessary to go very carefully over the patients movements 14 days previously to find out how infection may have been contracted. This includes enquiring into what food and drink may then have been consumed.

Incubation periods are never easy to remember and can vary in the same disease. They can be conveniently divided into three groups:

---

(1) *Very short incubation periods:* 2 hours – 18 hours

Staphylococcal toxin food poisoning
Salmonella food poisoning
Clostridium perfringens toxin food poisoning

---

(2) *Short incubation periods:* 2 to 7 days

Streptococcal infections, scarlet fever, puerperal infection, erysipelas, tonsilitis, Staphylococcal airborne infections – pemphigus neonatorum
Pneumonia
Diphtheria
Influenza
Meningitis
Dysentery
Infantile gastro-enteritis
Paratyphoid
Anthrax
Gonorrhoea

---

(3) *Long incubation periods*: 10 to 21 days

Lassa fever	(usually 10 days)
Marburg disease	(usually 10 days)
Chickenpox	(usually 17–21 days)
Rubella	(usually 17–20 days)
Measles	(usually 12 days)
Whooping cough	(usually 14 days)
Mumps	(usually 17–20 days)
Typhoid	(usually 14 days)
Poliomyelitis	(usually 11–14 days)
Syphilis	(usually 18–21 days)
Infective hepatitis	(usually 18–45 days)
Rabies	(usually 10–42 days but occasionally up to 4 months)

Bacteriological or virological investigations are most important in all communicable diseases. They aim at: (i) confirming the diagnosis (ii) discovering which close contacts are also infected (carriers).

In airborne bacterial diseases, nose and throat swabs can be taken. In tuberculosis, sputum tests, both by direct examination and culture, should be carried out on patients.

In the *faecalborne diseases, specimens of faeces or rectal swabs of patients and contacts should always be examined.* In most outbreaks, it is usual to find some contacts who are infected without symptoms (carriers). In many cases the carrier state may only last a short time but, if the carrier works with foodstuffs, further infections may easily be caused.

Blood examinations are also carried out. In the early stages of typhoid fever a positive blood culture will be found, allowing a certain diagnosis to be made earlier than by any other method.

In virus disease, virus isolations may be possible—e.g. influenza and poliomyelitis. Another method is to examine the blood very early in the illness and then about six weeks later when a significant rise will be noted in antibodies. This test can be used for a retrospective diagnosis in such cases. Because of the longer time taken with virus isolation and these blood examinations, they are less helpful in investigations than with the bacterial diseases.

Carriers

A carrier is someone who is infected with a disease and is excreting bacteria or virus causing the disease without suffering from any symptoms. They are of two kinds:

1 **Convalescent carriers**. People who have had the disease but who, in their convalescence, still excrete the bacteria. An example is a patient who has had typhoid, is now better, but who still has typhoid bacteria in the

faeces. Such people are usually temporary carriers, harbouring the bacteria for only a few weeks, but a few become permanent carriers, and intermittently carry bacteria in their faeces all their life (chronic typhoid carrier).

2 **Symptomless carriers.** These are people who have never had any illness or any symptoms but who are carriers. In such cases, infection produces a sub-clinical attack without symptoms, and the carrier state follows. An example is given by typhoid, which shows all types of carriers, or poliomyelitis. Symptomless carriers can also be either temporary or permanent.

Types of carriers

Anatomically, carriers can be divided into:

(a) *Nasal carriers*
Streptococci. Diphtheria. Staphylococci.
(b) *Throat carriers*
Diphtheria. Meningococci. Streptococci.
(c) *Faecal carriers*
Typhoid. Poliomyelitis. Dysentery.
(d) *Urinary Carriers*
Typhoid.

A chronic typhoid faecal carrier excretes typhoid bacilli in the faeces *intermittently*. Usually the faeces are positive for two weeks then negative for three to five weeks and then positive again. Because of this, repeated faecal examinations in typhoid are necessary otherwise a chronic carrier could be missed because the examination was carried out during a period when no bacteria were being excreted.

Special screening tests

X-rays form an important part of the investigation in an outbreak of tuberculosis.

Detailed methods of preventing communicable diseases

Airborne infections

Streptococcal infections

These include such varied diseases as scarlet fever, erysipelas, puerperal pelvic infection, tonsillitis, cellulitis and septicaemia. The usual method of infection is from either a case or unsuspected case, or from a nasal or throat carrier. It is also important to realize that the same type of streptococcus may cause scarlet fever in one patient, tonsillitis in another and even puerperal pelvic infection if a woman recently confined is infected. A careful search should always be made to discover any infections and, among very close contacts, a search for nasal carriers by examining bacteriologically nasal swabs is always worth while. Throat swabs are less useful.

In special problems such as the avoidance of puerperal infections, very great care must be taken to ensure that aseptic conditions are always maintained during and after confinement. *No midwife with a nasal or throat infection should ever be allowed to attend a mother in her confinement.* The midwife in such circumstances must remain off duty until better and until bacteriological examinations of her nose and throat are normal. If an unexpected streptococcal puerperal infection occurs, the nasal and throat swabs of all who attended the birth must be examined to make certain that none of them is a carrier.

Some of the most dangerous infections that can follow surgical operations are streptococcal ones. The stringent preventive measures taken in all surgical theatres to ensure aseptic conditions, including preparation of patient's skin, and theatre aseptic techniques, are all examples of preventive measures to reduce the chance of streptococcal infections.

In certain serious accidents, it may be impossible to prevent infection gaining access into a patient's tissues. In such cases, prophylactic treatment with chemotherapy and antibiotics is started as a further preventive measure.

Staphylococcal infections

Some of the most dangerous neo-natal cross infections in the nursery units of maternity hospitals are caused by penicillin-resistant staphylococci (pemphigus neonatorum). Preventive measures include:

(a) early recognition to enable the case to be promptly removed from the unit,

(b) strict barrier nursing techniques after the first case has been diagnosed,

(c) early discharge of mothers and babies so that time for cross infection is kept as short as possible,

(d) in those outbreaks which are not immediately controlled, the stopping of new admissions so that the chain of infection is closed.

Diphtheria

Immediately a case of diphtheria is diagnosed and removed to hospital, an investigation is started to discover the source of the infection. Nasal and throat swabs of close contacts (members of family and class mates) should be taken. Other members of the family are excluded from school until bacteriological tests are completed and also other members of the family are excluded from work if there is a risk of spread, e.g., a food handler.

Daily visits should be paid to the family by a health visitor or environmental health officer to check that no one has developed an illness as it is not only important to prevent the disease but to diagnose it early, when treatment is so much more effective. Other children in the family and close contacts should be given a booster immunization and those who have never been immunized should be given their first immunizing dose.

If any of the contacts is found to be a carrier, *a virulence test* must be carried out on the diphtheria bacteria isolated. A minority of these are avirulent—incapable of producing diphtheria. No carrier should be implicated as a possible source of infection until he has been confirmed to be carrying virulent diphtheria bacteria.

Any contacts who develop early suspicious signs should be given immediately a protecting dose of diphtheria antitoxin. An early small dose of such antitoxin is of great importance in reducing the severity of attack. The main method of *preventing diphtheria* is to see that *as many young children as possible are fully immunized* against the disease. Although it is hoped that the percentage of young children immunized will exceed 90 per cent, it is essential to see it never falls below 70 per cent for, below this figure, there is always a risk of an outbreak of diphtheria.

Tuberculosis

Although there has been a dramatic fall in the number of people developing pulmonary tuberculosis, 5859 cases occurred in England and Wales in 1981 (3627 men and 2232 women). This shows that tuberculosis is still a problem in this country.

Tuberculosis is usually diagnosed and treated by the chest physician at the chest clinic which is a specialized outpatient department. In some districts specially trained health visitors called *tuberculosis visitors* carry out the preventive health work with patients in conjunction with the chest physician. Most of this work involves home visiting.

The majority of cases of tuberculosis today are caused by direct infection from one human being to another by droplet (airborne) infection. The control and prevention of tuberculosis depends on:

(a) *Tracing of infection*
Tuberculosis does not spread like measles by chance, short-lived contact,

but follows fairly long and continued repetitive contact such as that which occurs among the members of the same household, classroom or office. When any new case occurs, it is essential to search *for the cause of the infection* among close contacts.

Arrangements are made to examine all members of the same family and household or members of the same office or classroom. In all instances, 'examination' must include a chest X-ray of all adults over the age of 15 years and, for children under this age, a tuberculin skin test and an X-ray for any found to be positive. It is most important that every effort is made to make certain that *every close contact* is examined. This is because the cause of the infection could be in someone who may have slight symptoms but may be afraid to have an X-ray. Because of the great preponderance of tuberculosis infection today in men over the age of 45, particular attention must always be paid to X-raying them. It is important to realize that a person may have a heavily infected sputum and be a most likely cause of infection and yet be able to carry on a normal life. Therefore, the *absence of any symptoms should never be used as an excuse to dispense with an X-ray.*

(b) *Steps to reduce the chance of infection*

(i) *Sputum disposal*

Every patient must be taught how to dispose safely of any sputum. Although it is hoped that in every patient the disease will be rendered quiescent, it is just possible that they may develop a transitory positive sputum from time to time and it is most important that, if this does occur, disposal of sputum is carried out carefully.

Expectoration of sputum should always be into a plastic sputum bottle containing a small amount of sterilizing fluid. This sterilizes the sputum after twenty minutes and also reduces its viscous and sticky nature, making disposal easier. The contents of each sputum bottle should be washed down a water closet *and never brought into the kitchen.* Each sputum bottle should have a plastic screw top (not metal as the sterilizing solution reacts with metal).

(ii) *Housing*

Overcrowded housing and sleeping accommodation produces conditions favouring the spread of this disease. No patient should ever sleep in the same room as another member of the family. The one exception is where the patient is a married person; in this case the couple can share the same room but should have twin beds. It is most important that *no parent who has had tuberculosis should ever sleep in the same room as a child.* Equally, no child with tuberculosis should share a room with other children.

If the house of the patient is not large enough to allow the patient to have a separate bedroom, *immediate rehousing is essential* to avoid infection spreading through the family. Most local authorities have special priority housing schemes which enable patients to be rapidly rehoused before further infection occurs.

(iii) *Occupation*

No person who has tuberculosis should be employed in an occupation in which there is a chance of spreading the disease if a relapse occurs. This means work should not be undertaken in the food trade or in close association with young children under the age of 12 years, such as teaching or nursery nursing. Consequently, no person is allowed to enter training to be a teacher unless he has a clear chest X-ray. Periodic check-ups for teachers are also encouraged. Likewise all staff employed in childrens' homes or nurseries should always be X-rayed before commencing their employment.

It is illegal for a person with open tuberculosis to be employed in the food trade.

(iv) *Follow-up*

Careful follow-up of all patients must be carried out for five years after infection. This follow-up should be both at a chest clinic and by home visits to ensure that social factors at home have not deteriorated. If this occurs, a relapse in health is more likely.

In follow-ups, careful note is made of the level of nutrition for it is known that if this is defective a relapse is more likely to occur.

It is wise for home visits to be paid at least *once in six months* even when the patient is quiescent. In women patients, this will ensure that any pregnancy will be known to the tuberculosis visitor before full term.

Pregnancy in a patient whose tuberculosis is controlled is likely to do no harm but it is essential that everything is done to help the mother meet this extra challenge. Delivery should take place in hospital and arrangements should be made for her to have a prolonged convalescence after delivery. The baby must be vaccinated immediately with BCG. If the problem is known early in pregnancy, before six months, it is usually possible to make satisfactory arrangements for the care of the baby and family. But if the problem is only discovered in the puerperium, the mother may ignore the convalescent period to look after her family and baby, and in this way, risk permanent damage to her health and, perhaps, spread of infection in her family.

With modern drug therapy, it is usual for the chest physician to treat early cases at home on chemotherapy. However, recent research has shown that in some of those treated at home, the patient fails to take drugs regularly. This means that full benefit will not be obtained from his treatment and there is a greater risk of drug resistance developing.

(c) *Immunization of those at risk*

The ingestion of live virulent tubercle bacilli by anyone may, or may not, result in a recognizable clinical infection of tuberculosis. In many instances, the individual has sufficient resistance to prevent a clinical infection occurring. In all cases, however, a skin sensitivity develops.

If later a minute quantity of old tuberculin is injected into the skin of such a person, a sharp reaction or flare occurs. This is called a Mantoux positive skin test or tuberculin positive test. It means that, at some time in the past, the person has been in contact with live tubercle bacilli. All such individuals should be X-rayed, as occasionally a latent infection will be found. If no disease is discovered it can be assumed that there is enough immunity to resist infection. In this way, the tuberculin test, although one of hypersensitivity, can be used as an indicator of immunity.

A negative tuberculin test occurs in people with no special sensitivity. All newborn babies are tuberculin negative, and the change to positive only occurs after subsequent infection.

Immunization using BCG vaccination should be offered to all negative reactors in the following groups:

1   all family contacts of cases
2   all medical students and nurses
3   all schoolchildren aged 10–13 years
4   children of immigrants in whose communities there is a high incidence of tuberculosis irrespective of their age.

(d) *Detection of unknown infections by mass X-ray*
There is no doubt that the main danger of spreading tuberculosis comes *from undetected cases who are sputum positive* but as yet undiagnosed. In some cases, the disease can become so chronic that such a patient may be infectious for many years without anyone discovering this fact. Such a case can infect numerous other people with whom contact is made and can be a serious menace.

Once diagnosed and discovered, the danger can quickly be minimized both by treatment and the other preventive measures mentioned. *Mass radiography* plays an important part in discovering these unknown cases. Each year about 27 per cent of the new cases of tuberculosis are discovered by this method.

Mass radiography consists of taking an X-ray photograph of the chest using a small film, either 35 mm, 70 mm, or 100 mm. This film is projected on to a screen and about 95 per cent of those X-rayed in this way can be cleared on this small film, while 5 per cent are recalled for a large film on which final diagnosis is made. Recall may be for technical reasons, such as a bad film, as well as any doubts about diagnosis.

Mass radiography can be used either:

(a) to screen contacts in the investigation of a local outbreak;
(b) in special industrial surveys;
(c) in wide community surveys;
(d) to allow general practitioners to refer doubtful cases;
(e) in special age surveys.

All are valuable but the widespread community survey has to be very carefully organized to be of any real use, and with the smaller amount of tuberculosis present today in the UK the mass survey is no longer worthwhile.

In the past, very successful surveys were carried out in Glasgow, Edinburgh and Liverpool in 1957–9 when 76–80 per cent of the population over the age of 15 years were X-rayed. The results of all these surveys were similar and large numbers of unsuspected active pulmonary tuberculosis cases were found. These results are very interesting and are now given below because they demonstrate the marked variation between the incidence of tuberculosis in both sexes at different age groups which are still present today. The Liverpool figures are typical:

Table 7.1 1959 Mass X-Ray Campaign, Liverpool
Acute cases per 1000 X-rayed

	15–24 *years*	25–34 *years*	35–44 *years*	45–59 *years*	60 + *years*
Males	0.9	2.5	2.6	4.4	5.5
Females	2.0	2.7	2.5	1.3	0.8

Total acute cases: 2.41 cases/1000 X-rayed. There is evidence that this age incidence is still present today and that the main problem of infection at present is still in the middle-aged and elderly men. In an attempt to overcome this, special age mass X-ray surveys have been carried out in which men over 45 years of age are X-rayed.

Measles, whooping cough, mumps and german measles

The prevention of most of these diseases depends more on postponing infection by active immunization in cases of whooping cough, measles and, in girls, german measles. Occasionally in measles or german measles passive immunization is used when an attack would be more dangerous than usual (either a young child under 1 year of age or, with rubella, a pregnant woman during the first three months of pregnancy). See Chapter 6 for immunization details.

There is no certain way to prevent infection of these airborne infections by isolation as they all are infectious in their earliest stages often before the diagnosis can be made.

Faecal-borne infections

Typhoid and paratyphoid fever

Typhoid fever can be spread by:

(a) water
(b) food

Paratyphoid fever is spread by food.

Prevention. The prevention of typhoid and paratyphoid depends on:

(a) full immediate investigation of cases to discover the cause

(b) control of chronic carriers

(c) food control including sampling at docks, pasteurization of milk supplies and ice cream, prohibition of infected shell-fish

(d) environmental hygiene

(e) immunization of holiday visitors to certain countries where the risk of infection is high e.g. Italy, Yugoslavia, Portugal, Spain and Africa.

In both diseases, infection is introduced into water or food by another human being who is either suffering from the disease or is a carrier.

Most infections result from carriers. The majority of cases traced in England and Wales are contracted abroad. For instance, in 1981, 254 infections were traced and of these 224 were contracted abroad. Any person who is a carrier and who handles food of any description or who is employed by water supply departments can be most dangerous.

For this reason, whenever a case of typhoid fever occurs, a complete investigation must be carried out immediately to find the cause of infection. A careful history is taken to find out what food was eaten by the victim and close contacts at the time of infection. This means inquiry at the start of the incubation period, fourteen days before the first symptoms in typhoid and seven days in paratyphoid fever.

Immediate stool examinations must be carried out on all close contacts and especially on all the kitchen personnel. If a carrier is discovered, the typhoid bacteria must be identified and typed by *phage typing*. It is possible to divide typhoid and paratyphoid bacilli into a *number of different types*. These are then compared with the type causing the outbreak. If the types are dissimilar, then the carrier could *not* have caused the outbreak. If the type is the same, the carrier *could* have been responsible. The discovery of a carrier of the same type does not prove the cause and further investigations must be undertaken.

The large typhoid outbreaks of the past were mainly water-borne due to water supplies being infected. In this country, the Croydon outbreak of 1937 involving 290 persons was the last large water-borne outbreak. This outbreak was caused by a urinary carrier among the workmen carelessly contaminating a deep well which formed part of Croydon's water supplies.

Careful methods of sewage disposal and purification and sterilization of water supplies which are universal in this country have reduced the likelihood of any further water-borne outbreaks in this country.

But every case must be carefully investigated to ensure that the cause is found. Omitting to do this could lead to a serious spread as was seen in the disastrous Zermatt water-borne outbreak of typhoid fever in 1963 resulting in 434 cases.

Food supplies may be infected by carriers. For this reason all known cases of *typhoid or paratyphoid are very carefully followed up* with fortnightly stool examinations *for at least six months or longer to make certain that they do not become chronic carriers.* About 5 per cent of all typhoid cases become chronic carriers and intermittently excrete typhoid bacilli, usually in their stools but occasionally in their urine. Animals are not a source of typhoid although some paratyphoid cases have been traced to infection in cows.

Once a chronic carrier is diagnosed, a careful check is kept on the occupation undertaken and other members of the family. No chronic typhoid or paratyphoid carrier is allowed to be employed in the food trade or to work in a kitchen or place where infection could be passed on. Members of the family of a carrier must be protected periodically by immunization with TAB vaccine.

In 1945 a serious outbreak of typhoid fever was caused in Aberystwyth by home-made ice cream being infected by a chronic carrier. Now, by law, all ice cream must be pasteurized, a heat process which kills any typhoid bacilli present.

In 1964 an extensive outbreak of typhoid fever occurred in Aberdeen. Over 400 cases occurred with 5 deaths. The most probable cause was a can of corned beef which contained typhoid bacillus. It is thought that the typhoid bacillus gained entry to the can after it had been sterilized. This probably occurred by the tin being cooled by contaminated unchlorinated river water.

To prevent any possible recurrences, it is essential that all water used for cooling in any canning process should be pure chlorinated water.

Food poisoning

The main causes of food poisoning are:

(a) *Chemical causes:* Tin, antimony
(b) *Bacterial toxin food poisoning*
  (i) *Staphylococcal* toxin
  (ii) *Clostridium perfringens* toxin
(c) *Salmonellosis*

Incidence. In England and Wales in 1981, 9925 cases of all types of food poisoning were traced, the majority being caused by various *Salmonella* bacteria.

All cases of food poisoning must be immediately and fully investigated, to discover, if possible, the cause. This investigation, if successful, will normally suggest ways and means of avoiding a recurrence.

Chemical food poisoning is only likely to occur when completely unsuitable containers (such as those made from galvanized iron) are used in which to cook foods.

(i) *Staphylococcal toxin food poisoning* results in foodstuffs being infected with certain strains of *Staphylococcus aureus* which, on multiplication within the foodstuff produce an *enterotoxin*, a poison acting upon the stomach. An interval of at least 12 hours must occur between infection of the food and its being eaten to allow sufficient toxin to be produced to lead to food poisoning.

Staphylococci usually contaminate foods from either a skin or nasal lesion in a food handler. They do, however, also attack the skin of animals and, in the cow, may lead to a staphylococcal infection of the udder with subsequent contamination of the milk.

Once staphylococcal food poisoning toxin has been produced in any foodstuff, it is *very difficult to destroy by heat as it is heat stabile*. This means that even boiling a foodstuff already contaminated with toxin would only destroy a very small and insignificant amount of that toxin.

As staphylococci are usually present in the noses of 10 per cent of people, this food poisoning can best be avoided by ensuring that all foods are:

(a) either eaten within an hour or two of preparation;

(b) if kept are always stored in cool, refrigerated conditions which are too cold for bacterial multiplication (toxins are produced only by bacterial multiplication);

(c) prepared under the cleanest conditions possible. This means that a high degree of personal hygiene is important. Hands must be frequently washed and habits avoided which would encourage transfer of staphylococci from the nose and mouth of the food handler to foodstuffs.

Great care must be taken to prevent any food handler who has an acute or chronic skin infection, infected cut, boil or paronychia from handling food. Legal regulations recommend *all infected cuts must be covered with waterproof dressings* to avoid contaminating foodstuffs. It is even more satisfactory to exclude from food handling any person so infected.

(ii) *Clostridium perfringens (Cl. welchii) toxin food poisoning* is less severe than staphylococcal toxin poisoning.

The toxin, which is also heat-stabile, is produced by multiplication of *Clostridium perfringens*, a spore-bearing anaerobic bacterium which also can cause gas gangrene. The spores of this bacteria are widespread—in soil and often in faeces. However, being an anaerobic bacterium, it will only multiply in the absence of oxygen. For this reason, it mainly produces food poisoning in meats or in stews and soups made by long standing low temperature simmering.

Prevention. Spores of *Clostridium perfringens* are found in many meats and therefore inevitably will gain access to kitchens. Infections with this type of food poisoning will only be avoided if the following rules are strictly observed:

(a) avoid precooking of meats

(b) avoid storing any food between 49°C and 10°C for more than 3 hours

(c) if meats have to be precooked, it is essential that they are rapidly cooled and maintained below 10°C in a domestic refrigerator.

(d) care must always be taken when gutting animals such as rabbits to avoid contamination of the flesh with faeces from the intestine (which will be likely to contain large quantities of spores of *Clostridium perfringens*).

Salmonellosis

Salmonellosis is usually the commonest type of food poisoning, and is an infective gastro-enteritis in which the small intestine is attacked by one of the salmonella bacteria, producing an acute inflammation. There are over 1000 serotypes but the commonest is *Salmonella typhimurium* which is responsible for 40 per cent of cases. *Salmonella enteritidis* and *agona* are the next commonest types found in the United Kingdom.

Method of spread. There are 6 main sources of salmonellosis:

1   human cases and carriers
2   domestic animals and rodents
3   eggs of ducks and hens
4   pigs
5   chickens
6   untreated raw milk

Any one of these sources may lead to contamination of food but fortunately a very heavy infection is necessary to lead to a salmonella food poisoning and this means that usually there is a history of incorrect method of storage of the food, e.g., the foodstuff has been stored for more than 12 hours at normal room temperatures and not refrigerated temperature – this allows rapid bacterial multiplication which will not occur at cold refrigerated temperatures. In addition it is wise to avoid duck eggs even in cooking.

Whenever an outbreak of salmonella food poisoning occurs, a complete investigation must take place to find if possible the cause of the infection.

A particular search for faecal carriers should always be made among all kitchen personnel and all should have their stools bacteriologically examined. If any carrier is found, it must not be assumed that he or she is necessarily the cause, for such a carrier may also have been infected in the outbreak. All carriers must stop handling food immediately and not do so again until they have been cleared. The carrier state usually lasts only a few weeks and it is unusual for it to become chronic.

Any foodstuff, which is precooked and then stored for a lengthy period before consumption, such as cooked and prepared meats, may be dangerous if storage has been faulty and the food has become infected. Naturally infected foods can also cause trouble. For example, serious outbreaks of food poisoning have been traced to heavily contaminated eggs and coconut products imported from abroad but fortunately an effective heat treatment has been devised.

Prevention. It will be seen that all salmonella food poisoning can best be avoided with:

(a) extreme care being taken in preparation of food, and with personal hygiene among food handlers. This reduces the chances of a carrier accidentally contaminating any food.

(b) all food prepared being eaten immediately. Any left over food should be thrown away. In this respect, it is most undesirable to prepare a sweet today for lunch tomorrow, unless stored in a refrigerator.

(c) where food, such as meat pies, is stored for a lengthy time, it must be stored at low temperature, below 4°C—preferably in a refrigerator.

(d) gamma radiation from a cobalt-60 source being used to destroy salmonellae in frozen whole egg, coconut, imported meats and animal feeding stuffs.

(e) pasteurization of liquid milk. Only 3 per cent of the population in the UK now drink untreated raw milk but, in all reported cases of salmonella food poisoning, 6.9 per cent are associated with the consumption of such milk.

Dysentery

The bacterial dysentery caused by *Shigella sonnei* (often called Sonne dysentery) is the commonest form of dysentery in this country. It is usually a mild, short-lived gastro-enteritis which is only serious in young babies or debilitated elderly persons.

Sonne dysentery is spread by direct contamination from person to person. In a closed community, such as a ward or nursery, it spreads slowly at first but, as soon as a substantial proportion of persons are infected, it spreads more quickly.

The best method to avoid outbreaks is:

(a) to diagnose dysentery early,
(b) to isolate all cases and carriers.

This is especially important in day nurseries and hospital wards. All cases of diarrhoea must be *bacteriologically examined* (stool specimens) to make certain that any early cases are identified—there is always a proportion of symptomless carriers among close contacts but usually they are carriers only for two to three weeks.

By careful investigation and isolation of cases and carriers, serious outbreaks will usually be avoided. If, however, a widespread outbreak has been allowed to develop, isolation will achieve little. The aim should, therefore, always be to diagnose the first cases and this can only be done if it is a rule to submit routinely for bacteriological examination stools of all patients who develop any diarrhoea, however mild or transient.

Infantile gastro-enteritis

This is a general term used for any severe gastro-enteritis in young infants. The exact cause of some outbreaks is often uncertain but in others infection has been traced to certain pathogenic strains of *Escherichia coli* including 0 26, 0 55, 0 111, 0 125, 0 126, 0 127, 0 128 and 0 229. Many enteroviruses (ECHO and Coxsackie B viruses) have also been identified as causes.

The virus responsible for many attacks of infantile gastro-enteritis can be identified by use of the electron microscope. Serologically the virus which unfortunately has been given many different names including reovirus-like agents, orbivirus, rotavirus and duovirus, is related to the virus of calf diarrhoea. As soon as the problems of culturing this virus in vitro are overcome it is hoped it will be possible to develop a prophylactic vaccine.

Prevention. These attacks can best be prevented by complete investigation when they occur and by arranging for all young infants to spend as little time as possible in hospital or residential nursery units. There is no doubt that many attacks result from cross infection—infection spreading rapidly from infant to infant in a ward. It is therefore most important that any infant with diarrhoea *is isolated immediately* and that *no child with a history of diarrhoea is ever admitted to a clean infants' ward* but straight into the *isolation unit*.

Once infection has occurred, especially the serious type of gastro-enteritis that occasionally attacks a nursery unit of a maternity ward, new admissions should be stopped and the ward emptied as soon as possible by discharging mothers and babies home early. In this way, the chance of widespread infection is reduced.

Attempts to control the spread of infantile gastro-enteritis by strict barrier nursing nearly always fail, probably because of the intensity of infection and the rôle infected dusts play in spreading the disease.

Encouragement of breast feeding can do much to reduce the incidence of infantile gastro-enteritis and every effort should be made to keep breast feeding going if the infant develops an illness. If the baby must enter hospital his mother should also be admitted so that breast feeding may be maintained.

Poliomyelitis

Poliomyelitis has the most well-defined seasonal incidence of any known communicable disease, for outbreaks in this country always occur in late summer and early autumn, in August, September or October. For this reason, there is only a serious risk of epidemic spread in these months. Fortunately following widespread immunization with oral poliomyelitis vaccine, the disease in the U.K. has become very rare.

Poliomyelitis is a faecal-borne disease which is spread by direct contact from person to person usually living in the same household. Although infected, the majority of close contacts show no symptoms and only rarely does clinical poliomyelitis result.

When a case of poliomyelitis occurs, it is therefore important that, as far as possible, the members of the same household are segregated from the general population. Child contacts should certainly be kept away from school for at least three weeks. By isolating the family as far as possible, the chance of spreading infection is reduced.

In addition, as soon as any case occurs, immediate immunization using oral poliomyelitis vaccine should be given to:

(a) all contacts at home, work or school

(b) all people living within an approximate radius of a quarter of a mile from the patient.

This not only serves to boost their immunity but also blocks the entrance of 'wild' or epidemic virus into their intestines and thus will help reduce the chance of further infection.

Household contacts should also be placed under surveillance for three weeks. They should be visited by a health visitor daily to check their temperature and whether they have any symptoms. If any abnormality is noted, then the contact should be put to bed immediately and kept as quiet as possible. This is important because *violent exercise in the patient showing the earliest signs of poliomyelitis can result in a severe attack*. As a further precaution, no close contact of a case of poliomyelitis should be allowed to indulge in strenuous exercise for three weeks. Close family contacts should, therefore, not go on walking tours or any similar activities at this time.

Restrictions among the general population regarding swimming baths are probably useless in preventing the spread of poliomyelitis. However, swimming is a fairly violent form of exercise and should be avoided for three weeks among close family contacts.

As already explained, the most valuable preventive measure against poliomyelitis is to make certain that as high a proportion as possible of people under 40 years of age are completely immunized against the disease using oral Sabin vaccine.

Cholera

Although classic cholera last appeared in epidemic form in the United Kingdom in 1866, recently there have been a number of outbreaks in westernized countries from the new El Tor strains.

The last two cases occurred in England in 1977. The first was an Iraqui man who developed the disease a few hours after his arrival from Bagdad. The second case was an English woman who developed acute vomiting and diarrhoea two days after return from a holiday in Turkey. Both were found to be infected with *Vibrio cholera* biotype El Tor serotype Ogawa. No secondary cases occurred. Modern rapid air travel facilitates the spread of this disease which has a short incubation period of 2–3 days.

Contamination of water supplies is the classic method of spread but flies can also be responsible if sewage disposal methods are crude. Direct spread from food handlers who are carriers is also a possibility.

El Tor cholera remains in the stools of cases for at least 14 days and occasionally for up to three months.

Prevention. This mainly depends on purification of water supplies and safe disposal of sewage. In epidemics, water and milk must be boiled (unless already pasteurized) and careful segregation of all patients arranged with terminal and concurrent disinfection.

Active immunization should be arranged for those at special risk (doctors and nurses) and for travellers to countries where the disease is epidemic. Immunization provides about 50 per cent protection for a short period and revaccination is advisable every 6 months. Results, however, have been disappointing against the El Tor type of vibrio.

Infective Jaundice

This disease is notifiable and approximately 9834 cases were recorded in England and Wales in 1981. About 60 per cent are children and in most outbreaks it is usually possible to trace a number of causes without clinical jaundice.

There are three types of infectious jaundice—hepatitis A, hepatitis B and hepatitis nonA/nonB. The notification figures do not distinguish between these types but the steady fall in notifications during the last ten years is probably due to a reduction in the number of cases of hepatitis A.

Carriers of hepatitis B in the community can raise special problems. Certain patients, e.g. those on dialysis, are known to be at special risk of infection with hepatitis B.

Prevention. There is no method of active immunization but recently success has been observed by using immunoglobulin as a passive immunity. This resulted in a reduction of cases and also in a modification in the severity of the subsequent disease.

Direct spread—from animals

Anthrax

This is a rare disease usually caught by direct spread from the hide of an animal, from wool or from the bones of animals. For this reason, anthrax is only seen in people whose occupations bring them into contact with animals and animal products. The main groups of people at risk include dockers handling hides who occasionally develop anthrax, and wool sorters.

The prevention of anthrax depends on:

(a) special treatment of wool imports to kill any anthrax spores at a number of centres close to the mills.

(b) protective clothing being worn by persons handling hides and bones.

(c) immunization against anthrax for all associated workers (see page 92).

As a further safeguard, the dangers of anthrax are explained to all those working in occupations in which there is a danger of contracting the disease. Diagrams of early symptoms are prominently displayed so that if anyone develops the skin lesions of anthrax, it is more likely to be recognized and diagnosed early. All such workers also carry a special card to show to their general practitioners when attending so that the doctor knows of the special risk of contracting anthrax which their occupation carries.

The early diagnosis is most important as modern treatment can quickly cut short an attack of anthrax.

Leptospirosis

This disease is caused by *Leptospira icterohaemorrhagiae* and is primarily a disease of rats. Infections in man result from the skin being infected by water contaminated with rat urine and usually only occur among abattoir or sewage workers who are most likely to come into close contact with rats. All such workers should be warned of the dangers of infection and of the importance of a high standard of hygiene. It is especially important that they *avoid contaminating skin with water which may have been infected by rat's urine*. It is especially dangerous to walk barefoot in such places.

Brucellosis

In the UK *Brucella abortus* produces a disease in cattle which also can cause the illness of brucellosis in man.

Prevention depends on:

(a) eradication of the disease from animals
(b) pasteurization (heat treatment) of all milk supplies.

There is a Brucellosis Incentive Scheme operated by the Ministry of Agriculture, Fisheries and Food, who carry out the testing of herds and who maintain a national register of brucella-free herds. To qualify for entry a herd must show three clear blood tests at four-monthly intervals. Money incentives are then paid for each gallon of milk produced and for each breeding cow in a beef herd.

In any outbreak of brucellosis, the local authority can apply for a 'pasteurization order' under the Milk and Dairies (General) Regulations 1959 if a milk sample shows the presence of *Brucella abortus*. Milk from such a herd must then be sent for pasteurization.

Rabies (hydrophobia)

At present in the United Kingdom considerable concern is being shown about the dangers and problems of rabies because of the increase of this disease on the continent. Many different wild animals can be infected (including foxes, otters and rodents) but the vast majority of cases in wild animals have been traced to foxes (about 90–94 per cent in European countries). In fact an epizootic in foxes has spread during the last 10 years to France from Germany, Switzerland, Austria, Denmark and Belgium. About 75 per cent of all animal outbreaks on the continent have occurred among wild animals and the remainder among domestic animals. Dogs are most commonly affected in this group but cats and bovines are also infected.

Two imported cases of rabies occurred in the United Kingdom in 1975. Both cases had been bitten by rabid dogs before arrival in this country and although both received intensive treatment both died. Another case from abroad died early in 1977. In 1978, one death occurred in an immigrant from Pakistan.

Prevention. The virus of rabies is in the saliva of rabid animals. After a bite from a rabid animal, the virus spreads in humans to the central nervous system producing the characteristic symptoms. The disease is very dangerous with a high mortality and anyone who has been bitten by a rabid animal must be immunized (see page 92). The incubation period is usually about 2–6 weeks but in a few cases may be much longer.

Rabies Act 1974. Under this Act, there is a compulsory six months quarantine period for all animals entering the country. Effective precautions must also be taken against the transmission of the disease within quarantine kennels. All dogs and cats entering quarantine must be vaccinated on entry with a proved potency-tested inactivated vaccine; they must also be revaccinated after one month in quarantine to extend immunity.

Dogs and cats are allowed to enter Britain only at a limited number of ports. Animals landed illegally may be destroyed on landing and the Act provides severe penalties, including up to one year's imprisonment for offences against the orders under the Act.

Further orders provide for a wider range of measures to control any outbreak of rabies in Britain. These include destruction of foxes, controls on the movement of domestic pets and their vaccination, the seizure of strays and the banning of hunting, and cat and dog shows.

Prophylactic vaccination against rabies (see page 92) should be offered to all persons who in their work are at risk including:

1   those employed at quarantine kennels
2   those working in quarantine premises in zoos
3   agents who are authorized to carry such animals
4   those working in research and acclimatization centres where primates and other imported mammals are housed
5   those working in ports regularly importing animals.

Booster immunization should be given every 2–3 years.

Contact infection from animals or humans

Viral haemorrhagic disease

There are three viral haemorrhagic diseases—Lassa fever, Marburg disease and Ebola virus disease. Each is caused by viruses. Symptoms include extreme malaise, muscular pains and haemorrhagic macula-papula rashes. The mortality rate is between 25 and 30 per cent. Infection in Lassa fever occurs in two main ways:

1   by food and dusts contaminated by virus from the Nigerian rat—this is the usual method of infection in Nigeria;

2 by person-to-person infection in hospitals, and this is the most likely route of infection by which the disease could be spread in the UK. Marburg disease has mainly occurred in laboratory staff who have handled infected African green monkeys. Ebola fever can spread by contact with a patient's blood. The incubation period of viral haemorrhagic disease is 3–21 days.

Special precautions are now laid down to deal with suspected cases:

1 early diagnosis. Any fever in a recently arrived traveller from Nigeria should be investigated to exclude Lassa fever, by blood culture and isolation of the virus and by evidence of antibody development;
2 immediate removal of any cases to special isolation hospitals using special ambulances;
3 strict precautions for all nursing staff (spread has been traced to accidental inoculation by needles);
4 daily surveillance of close contacts for 21 days. Anyone developing pharyngitis should be isolated.

Barrier nursing usually is effective to prevent spread of infection unless there is a severe pneumonia when infection can spread by air-borne droplets.

Sexually transmitted diseases (venereal diseases)

These are spread by direct contact in sexual intercourse—one partner infects the other.

In syphilis (incubation period about three weeks), gonorrhoea (incubation period 2–5 days) and in non-specific urethritis (incubation period 10–28 days) the mechanism of infection is similar.

The prevention of sexually transmitted disease depends on:

1 complete and efficient diagnosis and treatment of all cases;
2 the searching out of suspected cases;
3 avoidance of casual or promiscuous sexual intercourse.

(1) Diagnosis, especially of gonorrhoea, is not simple in the female, and an infected woman can remain so for a lengthy period without necessarily realizing she is infected. In doubtful cases, hospital out-patient attendance is desirable so that bacteriological smears may be taken and blood tests examined.

Inexpert treatment by inexperienced doctors is most dangerous for it may lead to incomplete cure and suppression of symptoms. The danger of double infection, gonorrhoea and syphilis in the same patient must be excluded. This can only be ensured if all cases of sexually transmitted disease are investigated and treated by the special hospital unit provided.

(2) Whenever a case of sexually transmitted disease is diagnosed, a careful history should be taken and arrangements made for the *cohabiting partner to be medically examined as soon as possible.* To carry out this contact tracing, specially trained nurses and social workers are attached to all sexually transmitted disease departments. Their task is to trace the cohabiting partner wherever possible and persuade him or her to come to the clinic for a full examination.

(3) Better education is needed, so that all persons realize that only by self control and avoidance of casual sexual intercourse will such disease be avoided. It is especially important to realize that, *without bacteriological tests, it is impossible even for a doctor to exclude the possibility of such disease in any person.* This should be explained to young men who may otherwise be misled by older men into believing they can tell when a contact is, or is not infected.

During the past few years, there has been a change in the pattern of sexually transmitted diseases in the UK. There has been an increase in the number of non specific genital infections, genital herpetic infection and candidosis.

There was also a slight rise in the numbers of new cases of early syphilis but the total number of cases of gonorrhoea has fallen from 59 028 in 1977 to 57 847 in 1979 (England). There has however been a disturbing increase in the penicillin-resistant gonococci identified—mostly from infections imported into the UK.

8
Prevention of Non-communicable Diseases

With non-communicable disease, the greatest barrier to prevention is that so little is known about the causes of disease. Research into the causation is continually being carried out and the factors connected with the incidence of such diseases are slowly being unravelled. It is, however, a very complicated study as there is a multiplicity of factors involved. Even in diseases whose cause is as yet hardly understood, wide differences exist between the various social classes as shown on page 35, suggesting that the living conditions of the various social classes may increase or diminish the dangers of developing such diseases.

Sometimes important factors only come to light by a steady increase in a disease leading to greater and greater research which finally finds an important causative factor. An example of this is given by *cancer of the lung*, the increase of which has been shown to be *connected with increased cigarette smoking*. But as yet, research even in this instance has not discovered all the chemical factors in cigarette smoke which produce this carcinogenic effect. Another example is bladder cancer. Epidemiological studies have indicated that there was a higher incidence of bladder cancer among workers in the dyestuffs industry and indicated three aromatic amines, α-naphthylamine, β-naphthylamine and benzidine as potent carcinogens. Also it was found that antioxidants made from α- and β-naphthylamines were used frequently in rubber and cable industries. Since the use of α- and β-naphthylamines were banned bladder cancers in men, who entered the industries after this ban, have fallen although those employed before the ban still show a marked excess.

Prevention of non-communicable diseases can always be considered from two aspects:

(a) complete prevention of the disease ever occurring in any individual (primary prevention).

(b) prevention of deterioration or of relapses from a disease already existing (secondary prevention). This includes early diagnosis and an understanding of the social and occupational factors which predispose to further attacks of the disease. It is also important to remember that unless the correct treatment is carried out continuously in a chronic disease such as diabetes, then the finest diagnostic and treatment facilities will be wasted. In many instances, *correct treatment depends on understanding many of the social factors which can negate success.*

Ischaemic heart disease

The incidence of ischaemic heart disease increased markedly during the last 21 years (see Table 2.12, p. 33). Ischaemic heart disease, the clotting of blood in the coronary arteries supplying the heart muscle with blood, is usually associated with an atheromatous condition of the linings of the arteries in which tiny plaques of fatty material are laid down in the linings of these arteries making clotting more likely. Much research has been carried out throughout the world to discover what causes this atheromatous condition. Much has yet to be discovered but it is already clear that enormous differences in incidence of ischaemic heart disease occur throughout the world. For instance, the death rate from this condition in America is nine times that of Japan. France too has low rates while her neighbours are high, including England, Wales and Scotland.

Table 8.1   Deaths from ischaemic heart disease per 100 000 population 1979 (both sexes)

Japan	38.4
Spain	77.7
France	91.6
Switzerland	136.0
Italy	160.1
Netherlands	178.0
USA	294.3
England and Wales	326.7
Scotland	357.0
Sweden	398.2

The reasons for these differences are not completely known. The latest views are that a number of factors are probably important including:

1 high blood lipid levels
2 hypertension
3 cigarette smoking
4 genetic factors
5 physical inactivity
6 increase in body weight
7 diabetes
8 nervous stress
9 cold weather in older patients
10 the sex of the individual

The short heavier person is more prone to an *early* attack than the tall thin person. Regular exercise seems to have some protective effect and farmers and others leading active lives have a lower incidence than sedentary workers. There is certainly an endocrine factor which is probably responsible for the higher rate in younger men. Under the age of 45, the disease is eight times commoner in men than in women. After the menopause the rate in women increases until by the age of 70 it is equal to that of men.

Prevention. At present, there is no agreement about the exact steps which should be taken to avoid ischaemic heart disease. Some suggest that it would be wise to do a routine blood cholesterol test on all men aged 35 and that, in those in whom a raised level was found, a diet should be commenced in which animal fats are replaced by vegetable fats. Also, care should be taken to avoid overweight. However, many physicians feel that to do this would only worry many patients unduly and, in the end, more harm could be caused.

Further research is necessary to try and find the most important causes. Until this has been achieved, there is no doubt that the following simple rules are most helpful and likely to reduce ischaemic heart disease:

(a) avoid overweight at all costs;

(b) constant exercise, such as walking should be encouraged— probably daily exercise is much more useful than sudden bursts of exercise;

(c) do not smoke cigarettes. *However, if anyone stops smoking, these risks will fall to the level of the non-smoker within 48 hours.*

For the patient who has already had an attack of ischaemic heart disease, these simple rules are even more important, as well as the avoidance of sudden cold such as a sea bathe in cold weather.

The cancers

The true causative nature of cancers is, as yet, unknown. There are, however, many associated factors now recognized which are known to predispose to the development of cancers—most of these are connected with some chronic recurring form of irritation. It is known that various skin cancers can be caused by irritation from oils and sunlight and cancers of the tongue by the irritation of a clay pipe. It is likely that the association between cigarette smoking and lung cancer, and between atmospheric pollution and lung cancer, is of this nature. A clear connection has also been demonstrated between the development of liver cancers (hepatic angio-sarcoma) and exposure to monomeric vinyl chloride. The greatest dangers have been traced to men who open and clean the autoclave where vinyl chloride is polymerized.

It is not always appreciated how cancers vary in incidence between social classes. The following figure indicates this very clearly:

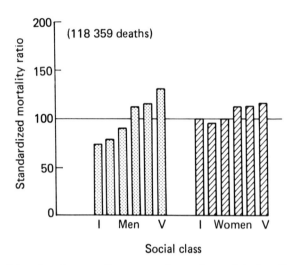

Fig. 8.1 Mortality from malignant neoplasms by social class for men and married women aged 15–64, England and Wales, 1970–2. (From *Occupational Mortality*, 1970–2, OPCS.)

Most cancers show their highest incidence in social class V and their lowest incidence in social class I. It is not known why cancer of the breast differs in this respect.

Prevention in cases of irritation can best be achieved by removing or avoiding the predisposing factor.

In other cases, the recognition and radical treatment of a very early precancerous condition can help to prevent the subsequent development of cancer.

Cancer of the cervix uteri

Cancer of the cervix uteri was responsible for the deaths of 2068 women in 1980 in England and Wales but this death rate has been falling. Table 2.13 (p. 35) shows the marked variation in the various social classes. Repetitive damage to the cervix uteri is a predisposing cause to this cancer and this is one of the reasons for a higher rate in social class V women who generally have larger families than women from social class I or II.

Prevention. There is now a widely used screening test (exfoliative cytology) which can detect a precancerous condition in the cervix. The technique of the test is simple. A vaginal speculum is passed and a direct smear is obtained from the cervix and examined histologically. If there are abnormal mitotic changes in the nuclei of the epithelial cells removed, a complete gynaecological examination should be carried out and a cone biopsy undertaken to find whether a precancerous cancer *in situ* exists. If these investigations confirm a precancerous condition, it is then usual to operate and remove the cervix (or complete uterus) before a dangerous invasive cancer develops.

Such smears are collected by general practitioners or at a special clinic. Regular testing in this way should be carried out on all women once every three years.

Cancer of the lung

The increase in cancer of the lung recently has been most dramatic. The disease has become commoner since the early part of this century, but the greatest increase has been in the last thirty years.

It is always difficult when comparing the incidence of any disease over a number of years to assess how much better diagnosis may be responsible—in other words, how much of the increase is apparent and not real. However, if the incidence of cancer of the lung is examined in England and Wales over the last thirty three years, 1947 to 1980, it is possible to ignore this diagnostic factor as, by 1947, widespread use of radiology and bronchoscopy was taking place in the diagnosis of lung lesions, and it is safe to assume the degree of diagnosis was similar. In this period of twenty-eight years, the number of deaths from cancer of the lung has more than doubled from 9204 in 1947 to 36 184 in 1982 (Table 8.3).

This increase is serious especially as cancer of the lung is difficult to treat effectively and usually results in the patient's death within $1\frac{1}{2}$ to 2 years of diagnosis in all but 5 per cent of cases. Prevention of lung cancer is one of the most serious problems facing medicine today. This is because cancer of the lung is easily the commonest cancer and it is unique, as it alone is the cancer which is increasing.

There are marked differences between the incidence of the disease in various countries (see table 8.2). However it will be noted that in all countries, cancer of the lung is commoner in men.

It will be noted that England and Wales is in the unenviable position of having the worst figures. This may be partly associated with additional climatic hazards.

Much research in various parts of the world has been carried out to investigate the factors associated with this great increase in cancer of the lung. All the various surveys in different countries have shown that more lung cancer patients are smokers of cigarettes than are the controls in the experiments. It has also been shown clearly that death rates from lung

Table 8.2   Deaths from Cancer of the lung per 100 000 population 1977 (both sexes).

	Males	Females
Japan	22.1	8.1
Australia	50.1	11.3
France	51.8	6.6
USA	63.1	18.6
Germany (Fed. Rep.)	69.0	10.0
Austria	74.6	14.3
Netherlands	91.6	7.4
England and Wales	111.6	28.9

cancer increase steeply as consumption of cigarettes increases. Heavy cigarette smokers have thirty times the death rate of non-smokers.

The Royal College of Physicians has studied the problem and clearly states that 'cigarette smoking is an important cause of lung cancer. If the habit ceased, the number of deaths caused by this disease should fall steeply in the course of time'.

Research in America has also shown that there are highly abnormal cells in the sputum of heavy smokers—cells which are showing many abnormal changes and may be precancerous. The interesting and encouraging feature is that, if smoking stops, then, within a short space of time, there is a diminution in the number of such cells in the sputum and finally they disappear altogether. This suggests that to give up smoking is to reduce the chance of developing cancer of the lung—a repeated finding reported from all surveys.

Table 8.3   Deaths from cancer of the lung, England and Wales

1947	9 204	1963	24 434
1951	13 247	1970	30 284
1955	17 272	1979	34 730
1959	21 063	1982	36 184
			(26 947 men, 9237 women)

As it is not possible to differentiate those people who will develop cancer of the lung, if they continue to smoke, the only certain and practicable way to prevent cancer of the lung is to reduce the amount of cigarette smoking. It is most important to discourage young people from starting the habit which has no real advantages and, as well as damaging health, is most costly.

Careful examination of Table 8.3 shows a definite steady upward trend. Women have not smoked for as long as men but today are rapidly becoming heavier smokers. Cancer of the lung used to be mainly a male disease but today the proportion of women who develop it, although smaller than men, is rising. *It is likely to continue to rise steeply unless smoking is reduced.*

No sensible person, who has studied the real facts could have any doubts about the connection between cigarette smoking and lung cancer. Yet, ever since the publication of the well known reports of the Royal College of Physicians in 1962, 1970 and 1983, cigarette consumption in this country has steadily increased and is now higher than ever before. As yet, although most adults have heard of the risks, they ignore them even to the extent of not discouraging their children from starting to smoke.

The problem is becoming increasingly important every year. Much more interest and encouragement is needed to teach people the dangers of smoking. More help could be given to those who wish to give up smoking by the setting up of anti-smoking clinics.

The Royal College of Physicians ended their reports by suggesting seven courses of action:

(i) more education of the public and especially schoolchildren concerning hazards of smoking.

(ii) more effective restrictions on the sale of tobacco to children;

(iii) restriction of tobacco advertizing;

(iv) wider restriction of smoking in public places;

(v) an increase of tax on cigarettes, perhaps with adjustment of the tax on pipe and cigar tobaccos;

(vi) informing purchasers of the tar and nicotine content of the smoke of cigarettes;

(vii) investigating the value of anti-smoking clinics to help those who find difficulty in giving up smoking.

Cancer of the breast

Cancer of the breast is an important cause of death in women. Table 2.13 (p. 35) shows that there is not much difference between the mortality among the different social classes in the UK. There is however a much wider range between the mortality in different countries as shown in Table 8.4.

Table 8.4 Cancer of the Breast death rate (females) per 100 000 population 1978

Japan	Greece	U.S.A	Netherlands	Denmark	England and Wales
6.5	19.6	31.0	36.0	40.7	46.9

Breast feeding is common in Japan and this fact may be partly responsible for the low death rate there. The high death rate in England and Wales emphasises the urgent need to prevent this disease as far as possible. The Standard Mortality Ratio, or SMR (1968 = 100), for 1979 for cancer of the breast was 110 showing that deaths from this cancer are increasing. The reduction in mortality from cancer of the breast is linked with early diagnosis. The type of cancer is also an important factor—the most rapidly spreading types being those which occur in pregnancy and lactation. Much cancer education today is directed towards explaining how important it is for women to palpate their breasts when taking a bath, and to report to their doctor at once if any form of lump is discovered, so that an investigation can be made immediately. Note that the survival rate seven years after treatment is 43.6 per cent (1978) and there is evidence that the earlier the treatment is started, the better the results.

Cancer of the stomach

The second commonest cancer in England and Wales is of the stomach. In 1982 10 211 people died from this disease (5978 men and 4233 women). It is interesting to note that in cancer of the stomach there is:

1 A well-marked variation in the social classes rising steadily from a SMR of 50 for class I to 153 for class V (Fig. 8.2).
2 A well-marked geographical association and the highest rates are in the rural areas of North Wales.

Fig. 8.2 Mortality from cancer of the stomach by social class for men aged 15–64, England and Wales, 1970–2. (From *Occupational Mortality*, 1970–2, OPCS.)

3   An association between chronic gastric irritation—chronic gastritis or even a previous gastric ulcer—and the subsequent development of a cancer.

The geographical variation which is so striking has stimulated much research to find out whether the residents of the rural areas of North Wales show special preferences for certain foods, but so far little has been found. A clue to the causation of this disease probably lies in its geographic and social class differences.

Cancer of the bladder

There are many more cases of cancer of the bladder in men than in women (in the ratio of 2.2 : 1.0). Reference has already been made (see page 121) to the incidence of cancer of the bladder in the rubber and cable industries due to exposure of workers to benzidine and naphthylamine-based derivatives.

There is also a marked difference in incidence in this cancer between different parts of the UK (see Table 8.5)

Table 8.5   Incidence of mortality from cancer of bladder
UK 1976 (SMR 1968 = 100)

	Females	Males
Northern Ireland	78	67
England and Wales	97	100
Scotland	136	105

Bronchitis

In England and Wales bronchitis was responsible for 18 874 deaths (13 124 men, 5750 women) in 1982. In addition it caused a great deal of invalidism in many sufferers and was responsible for much loss of working time in industry. Bronchitis has been called the 'English disease' as it is so common in this country compared with other countries of the world.

Our damp sunless winter climate may be connected with this increased incidence and the problem is made worse by atmospheric pollution which turns fog into poisonous smogs as the smoke and sulphur fumes become trapped within the fog. It is obviously impossible to alter the climate but two important preventive measures are possible to reduce the incidence and severity of bronchitis:

1   A reduction in cigarette smoking. There is no doubt that all smokers,
    and especially cigarette smokers, are much more often affected than
    non-smokers.
        Anyone with a tendency to *early bronchitis or asthma must
    stop smoking immediately.*
2   A reduction in atmospheric pollution. Much has already been
    achieved following the Clean Air Act 1956 whereby many areas were
    converted into smoke control areas in which it is illegal to burn
    ordinary coal which produces so much pollution. Because of financial
    restrictions this conversion has had now to be deferred.

Peptic ulceration

Peptic ulceration shows a marked variation in mortality between the
social classes (see Fig. 8.3).

There are other marked epidemiological differences between gastric

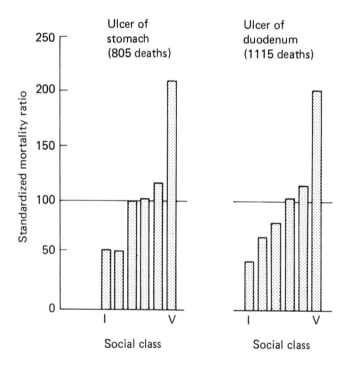

Fig. 8.3 Mortality from ulcer of the stomach or duodenum by social class for
men aged 15–64, England and Wales, 1970–2. (From *Occupational Mortality*,
1970–2, OPCS.)

and duodenal ulceration. Gastric ulcers are four times commoner in men than in women. But duodenal ulceration is more commonly associated with mental stress. There is a particular increase in the incidence of duodenal ulcer in professional persons such as doctors and lawyers who accept a considerable degree of personal responsibility.

There is often a strong association with the occupational regime followed by patients suffering from peptic ulcers. Those whose occupations do not allow them to have regular meals, such as long-distance drivers, can often trace lapses in their ulcer history to periods when irregular meals were usual.

The prevention of recurrence of peptic ulcers depends as much on being able to regulate, as far as possible, the life of the patient so that irregular meals and worry are avoided, as on the medical treatment of the condition.

Deaths from both gastric ulcer and duodenal ulcer are falling in men but rising in women.

Diabetes

This is a disease commoner in women than in men. Over 200 000 cases of diabetes have been diagnosed in the UK but the incidence may be considerably higher as there are always many mild undiagnosed cases (in 1961 a survey in Bedford with a population then of 61 000 brought to light 356 such undiagnosed diabetics).

The disease is really of two types:

1 The more serious diabetes seen in younger persons in which there is a strong heredity factor. In studies of such diabetes it has been shown that if one twin develops the disease the chance of the other also developing diabetes is five times greater in identical twins than in other twins.

2 The 'adult' type of diabetes which is a much milder disease usually controllable by diet. There is a higher incidence of adult diabetes in overweight persons. In the 1939–45 war less adult diabetes occurred and this was probably connected with less overnutrition due to food rationing. The avoidance of obesity is therefore an important preventive feature of adult diabetes (see below).

Another aspect of diabetes where prevention is possible, is *to ensure that treatment prescribed is properly carried out, by arranging for a health visitor to visit regularly all diabetic patients.* If the health visitor is attached to the diabetic clinic, she will be able to get to know the treatment prescribed for each patient. By visiting regularly, she can check whether the treatment is understood and is being followed and whether any early complications, such as peripheral skin lesions are present.

Adverse social conditions in the home can have a disastrous effect on the treatment of diabetes and this visiting can reduce difficulties at home. It also allows the physician treating the disease a means of discovering at an early stage any problems which the patient may have in treating the disease at home.

Obesity

Marked overweight is associated with an increased tendency to develop the following diseases:

(a) diabetes
(b) ischaemic heart disease and heart failure
(c) degenerative arthritis.

As the obesity increases, the expectation of life of the individual falls—it has been estimated that the expectation of life decreases by 1 per cent for every 1 lb. weight above normal.

Because of this clear association, much illness can be prevented by reducing the weight of persons who are excessively overweight. In particular, *it is most important that the tendency towards overweight is checked in the age group 35 to 50.* The aim should always be to keep the weight below average.

Three distinct types of obesity are:

1 'Hibernators' who are overweight persons who have adapted to low-energy diets so that dieting produces less and less effect. Such patients can now have their metabolic rate (and therefore their rate of weight loss) returned to normal under carefully controlled conditions in a metabolic ward.
2 The 'compulsive eaters' who form a large and well-recognized group whose obesity is entirely due to their continuously ingesting much larger quantities than they need. Any method which reduces the food intake of such patients will reduce their weight. Various strictly controlled dieting methods can be used but often fail eventually because of the tendency of such people to over-eat later. A novel and simple method is to fit such patients with a dental splint which forces them to stick to a milk-based diet. This has proved a satisfactory method for it prevents any return to uncontrolled eating at the end of any dietary regime.
3 The 'small' fat people whose energy requirements are very small because they have so little lean tissue. Such obese patients, who fortunately are a small group, are very difficult to treat and the condition may prove intractable once it has become firmly established.

Epilepsy

The problems created by epilepsy are:

(a) to find an effective treatment which will control the fits

(b) to help the patient to overcome the social disadvantages which too often follow epilepsy

(c) treatment must be continuous and always calls for much care and patience to ensure that the best combination of drugs is found

(d) unfortunately many stigmas are attached to the patient with epilepsy, mainly due to ignorance on the part of the public who mistakenly believe that it causes dangerous behaviour. Many such patients finds it essential to conceal their disease.

Often, much illness and many problems can be prevented by special care being taken in the rehabilitation of people with epilepsy. The question of stigma must never be ignored. By the better understanding, which follows social after-care and preventive work, it is often possible to prevent someone who suffers from epilepsy from losing his job, and to add stability to his life.

Much still requires to be done both individually with patients and collectively to educate the general public as to the true nature of this disease. Reference has already been made in Chapter 5 to the educational problems in epilepsy (see page 85).

Nutritional disorders

It is necessary for minute quantities of vitamins to be taken continuously by humans to maintain their health. A serious deficiency of vitamins (avitaminosis) will lead to the development of various deficiency diseases. A good sensible mixed diet will avoid any of the deficiency diseases in the adult. The following are the important vitamins:

Vitamin A (or its precursor). Found in liver, herring, eel, sardines, fish, liver oils, cheese, tomatoes, spinach and carrots. This vitamin is also introduced into most butters and margarines.

Vitamin B. Liver, lean meat, bacon and ham, wholemeal bread, oatmeal, nuts, peas and beans, rice-bran, yeast, marmite and bemax.

Vitamin C. Potatoes, hips and haws, brussels sprouts, tomatoes, oranges, lemons, grapefruit, watercress, asparagus tips, parsley, blackcurrants.

Vitamin D. Mackerel, herring, fish liver oils, salmon, eggs (yolk).

Deficiency diseases do not often occur in this country, although rickets was commonly seen 55–60 years ago.

Vitamin A deficiency

Vitamin A is essential for the proper health of epithelial surfaces and for the regeneration of visual purple in the retina.

A deficiency of vitamin A leads to:

(a) difficulties in night vision and eventually night blindness (an inability to see in very poor light);

(b) keratinization of the cornea and also to a hyperkeratosis of the skin.

Vitamin B deficiency

The vitamin B complex contains at least three important factors, *vitamin B_1, riboflavine*, and *nicotinic acid*.

Vitamin B_1 deficiency in an acute form is seen in tropical countries, as the disease *beri-beri*. In this country, vitamin B_1 deficiency is usually associated with chronic alcoholics who are taking a high carbohydrate diet with a very low intake of vitamin B_1. Symptoms are those of a peripheral neuritis.

There is a slight risk of vitamin B_1 deficiency in patients on special diets for gastric ulcer, coeliac disease or obesity, but this risk is well known and vitamin B_1 is invariably given to such patients.

Riboflavine deficiency in man shows itself as a dermatitis of the seborrhoeic type affecting skin around the nose and mouth. Riboflavine should always be given to patients on long courses of wide spectrum antibiotics to prevent a possible subsequent deficiency.

Nicotinic acid deficiency is a major factor in the production of the disease pellagra seen in the maize-eating communities of eastern Europe and Asia. Occasionally it is seen in this country in chronic alcoholism with steatorrhoea.

Vitamin C deficiency

This leads to scurvy, a disease in which bleeding occurs in mucous membranes. Until 170 years ago scurvy was the disease which plagued all sailors whose long voyages using dried foods meant invariably a deficiency of vitamin C. However, Lind discovered that the disease could be avoided by a daily ration of 1 oz. of lime juice. This was an important discovery and is said to have had the immediate effect of doubling the strength of the British Navy as it meant that no longer did ships have to return to port and release their crews every ten weeks. Although it was not then known why lime juice prevented scurvy, this is an excellent example of how a deficiency disease was prevented.

Today in this country there are two groups of people who are liable to suffer from vitamin C deficiency:

(1) *young infants.* All babies, being fed on either breast or dried milks, should always be given vitamin C additives. A convenient form is either orange juice or rose hip syrup;

(2) *old people living on their own* often neglect their diet and are commonly found to have a vitamin C deficiency on being admitted to hospital for some other cause. Occasionally signs of mild scurvy are found among old people living alone. This is most likely to be seen at the end of the winter. Preventive measures include arranging for the diet of the old person to be varied and to contain plenty of vegetables and fresh fruit. The simplest way to ensure this in old people neglecting their diet at home is to arrange for them to have 'Meals on Wheels' delivered to them at least three times a week or, if practicable, for them to attend a luncheon club (see page 251). In this way, it is possible to make certain that sufficient vitamin C is being supplied to them.

Vitamin D deficiency

Vitamin D deficiency leads to *rickets*, which is a disease of nutrition occurring in early childhood. Rickets is extremely rare today in this country. A few years ago, an increase in rickets was reported from Glasgow. This is a timely reminder that, if standards of nutrition fall in any area due, for instance, to increased unemployment, rickets can quickly follow.

In rickets, there is an interference with the normal mechanism of ossification of the bones. Irregular ossification occurs and this leads to various deformities.

Rickets has been largely eliminated from this country by the introduction of vitamin D additives in margarines and by the practice of making certain that all babies have vitamin additives, the importance of which is stressed by health visitors to mothers.

It is interesting to note that the rationing regime of the 1939–45 war, with its great emphasis on the importance of welfare foods such as orange juice and cod-liver oil, did much to educate the public of this country. The importance of a sound varied diet containing the necessary vitamins and also proper proportions of proteins, fats and carbohydrates was emphasized. Much health education work today in maternity and childhealth clinics concentrates on the importance of making certain that the diet is well balanced. This lesson is taught to all pregnant women, as women are particularly receptive to health education in pregnancy, and to all mothers regarding their young children. The lesson of good nutrition is continued in schools both by teaching and example.

Already the changes in nutrition have had an effect on the new generation of the children born in the last 25 years and it is estimated that on an average the school child today is at least 2 inches taller than his counterpart 30 years ago—a change solely brought about by better nutrition.

Goitre

Goitre is an enlargement of the thyroid gland and is usually seen in certain areas of the world, especially Switzerland, parts of France, Derbyshire and Somerset.

The cause of this enlargement is still uncertain but it has been found that the addition of a very small amount of iodine to salt (1 part in 100 000) has greatly reduced goitre in these areas and this is now the normal practice.

Fluoridation of water supplies and dental caries

The association between the amount of natural fluoride in water supplies and the amount of dental caries has led to much research into this question.

It is now clear that a level of 1 part of fluoride per million parts of water is sufficient to reduce significantly the amount of dental caries in children. Many countries of the world including America, Canada and New Zealand have now accepted this practice as a most useful preventive health procedure.

In this country, successful field trials have been carried out in certain areas and the Department of Health and Social Security has strongly advised water authorities to introduce this important preventive health programme. Approximately seven million people in England are now receiving fluoridated water supplies. Unfortunately ill-informed persons have attempted to prevent this advance because of the mistaken viewpoint that there may be danger in the practice. The Secretary of State for Social Services has repeatedly advocated wider use of fluoridation of public water supplies to prevent future generations of children losing their teeth through repeated attacks of dental caries. (See also p. 168).

Iron deficiency anaemia

Infants. A mild degree of anaemia is commonly present in all infants but this normally disappears on the introduction of a mixed diet. However, it is important to realize that, unless some form of iron is introduced into the diet, it may get worse if weaning is delayed. For this reason, it is usual to give small additional doses of iron in the diet to avoid further anaemia.

Adults. In adults iron deficiency anaemia to some extent is commonly present in women between ages of 20 and 50. It is probably due to:

(a) insufficient intake of foodstuffs containing iron
(b) loss of iron in bleeding in menstruation.

The prevention of this anaemia is to encourage a well-balanced diet with adequate proteins and vitamins. Once a degree of anaemia has been confirmed, large doses of iron are given by mouth.

Diseases connected with occupation

A number of diseases are caused by contact with various poisons, irritants and dusts. The prevention of such industrial diseases is the responsibility of the occupational health services.

Strict standards are laid down regarding the uses of all dangerous chemicals, solvents and gases in industry which could lead to illness. These include the following:

(a) dangerous metals—lead, phosphorous, mercury, arsenic, manganese, antimony, cadmium, chromium, nickel, copper, aluminium
(b) oils, pitch and tar
(c) dangerous gases—ammonia, benzol, carbon dioxide, carbon monoxide, carbon tetrachloride, chlorine, nitrous fumes, petrol, phosgene, sulphur dioxide, sulphuretted hydrogen, trichlorethylene
(d) dangerous solvents
(e) radiation hazards in industry.

Safety measures in industry come under the HM Superintending Inspector of Factories to whom all poisoning accidents must be reported. A full investigation is always carried out and wide publicity given to any important preventive method recommended.

Illnesses from industrial poisons vary greatly, from blood disorders to cancers of the skin and to occupational dermatitis. In some instances, such as workers who are continuously working with lead, regular routine blood tests must be carried out to make certain that no hidden changes are occurring in the blood which could be a sign of cumulative poisoning.

Some industrial dermatitis can be avoided by all workers having a medical examination *before* they start to work on hazardous jobs. In this way, it is possible to prevent certain susceptible people ever running these risks. This has been very useful in ensuring that persons with a previous or family history of dermatitis are never employed in a process in which determatitis is a hazard.

Prevention of dust diseases

The chronic inhalation of certain dusts eventually leads to the development of pathological lesions in the lungs. The most dangerous dusts are those containing minute particles of *silica or asbestos dusts.*

The term *pneumoconiosis* is used to describe diseases caused by these dusts. The industries in which dusts are hazards include a section of the coal-mining industry where extraction of coal includes mining in areas where silica dust occurs. The South Wales hard anthracite mines are a good example.

The level of pneumoconiosis (especially silicosis) was very high from such mines before preventive health measures were introduced. Silicosis is a fibrotic lung disease in which the lung tissue is slowly destroyed and replaced by fibrosis. Emphysema with loss of vital capacity follows, leading eventually to complete invalidism. Tuberculosis is a common complication.

Strict preventive measures now include:

(a) Regular medical examinations, including X-ray, of all men employed in any occupation in which pneumoconiosis is a risk.

(b) Immediate suspension from work of anyone found to be suffering from pneumoconiosis, including the earliest radiological signs, or from tuberculosis, together with the payment of a special financial benefit.

As well as these medical examinations, dust diseases can be prevented by:

(a) Replacement of a dangerous dust with a harmless one. An example is replacement of sandstone wheels for grinding metals by carborundum. Of course, this replacement is not possible in mining.

(b) Dust suppression by good general ventilation, by exhaust ventilation over the process, or by introducing a wet process in which dusts are kept to the minimum.

(c) Personal protection of workmen by the wearing of masks. This is usually only possible for short spells. General reliance should never be placed on workers wearing protective masks.

The inhalation of asbestos dust over a period of years leads to asbestosis. This disease is rather similar to silicosis, although tuberculosis is a rare complication. However, the *risk of cancer of the lung is greatly increased in asbestosis* and has been estimated to be at least ten times that of the general population.

The various preventive measures mentioned above have greatly reduced the risk of developing pneumoconiosis. They also reduce the seriousness of the condition if it occurs by removing the individual from the dusty occupation as soon as the earliest abnormal signs are discovered on X-ray.

Prevention of accidents

Increased attention has been paid recently to all forms of accidents both at work, in the home and on the road.

Traffic accidents

Motor vehicle and other traffic accidents are a major cause of accidental deaths—in England and Wales in 1982 5241 persons (3684 men, 1557 women) were killed in accidents on the roads. The introduction of compulsory seat belt legislation in early 1983, however, was followed by a dramatic fall in the injuries and deaths of drivers and front seat passengers, demonstrating the effectiveness of such preventive measures.

Industrial accidents

About 560 persons are killed every year at work—360 men and just under 200 women.

There are many contributory factors in occupational accidents, all of which are preventable. Accidents at work can be prevented by:

(a) Careful selection and training of personnel in the factory. Certain people are found to be 'accident prone'—that is, they are very liable to have accidents. Such people can sometimes be recognized early and steps taken to see that they are not placed in positions of danger.

(b) Complete investigation of all accidents. This is undertaken by the Chief Inspector of Factories who publishes an illustrated booklet every quarter, where the causes of accidents are analysed so that the reasons for the accidents can be pointed out, and similar catastrophes avoided.

(c) Good working conditions—good lighting, intelligent use of colours in factories, proper guarding of all machinery.

(d) Good discipline among employees including the wearing of protective clothing. In this country, there has been a great resistance to protective clothing—for instance, the wearing of steel helmets among building operatives. However, there are now signs that more protective clothing is being worn—certainly it can be decisive in preventing injury in the event of an accident.

Home accidents

Reference has already been made in Chapter 4, page 65, to the importance of preventing home accidents among young children.

There is a great deal of social class differential in mortality among children aged 1–14 as shown by the following table:

Table 8.6 Fatal accidents in childhood by sex and social class—(1–14 years)

				Social Class					Ratio
	I	II	III N	III M	IV	V	*All*	V/I
Boys	25.8	39	44.5	56.3	66.2	122	58.6	4.7
Girls	18.8	19	21.4	24.9	35.1	63.1	29.4	3.4
Sex Ratio	1.36	2.05	2.08	2.26	1.88	1.93	1.99	

Rates per 100 000 population

Source: *Occupational Mortality 1970–72* (OPCS)

The other age group which is particularly liable to home accidents is old people over the age of 65 years. Falls and falling objects are the main cause of their accidents. The extra dangers of accidents in the home for older people are shown clearly in Table 8.7 which gives details of such deaths by age and sex groups for England and Wales for 1972. It is important to note the larger numbers of deaths in old women compared with old men, a finding closely connected with the much larger numbers of older women in the community.

Table 8.7 Deaths from home accidents England and Wales 1972
(per 100 000 population)

Males aged				Females aged			
0–14	15–44	45–64	65+	0–14	15–44	45–64	65+
329	376	425	878	264	241	475	2371

These accidents can be prevented by:

1 Good lighting, especially on staircases, landings and passages.
2 Renewal of faulty equipment—worn carpets, broken stair rods, carpets not properly secured, trailing wires from electrical equipment, loose floor boards.
3 Ensuring that visual defects in the elderly are corrected by suitable spectacles
4 Better understanding by old people of the dangers of home accidents—more effective health education in this respect would help.

Prevention of mental illness

The exact cause of most mental illness is not yet fully understood. However, a great deal is already known about some of the factors related to its development. These include:

1 *Intrinsic* factors connected with the individual and particularly associated with

   (a) heredity
   (b) developmental factors.

2 *Extrinsic* factors to do with his occupation, home and life surroundings.

(1) *Intrinsic* factors are complicated. Hereditary factors are more of an inherited predisposition to develop mental illness than being born with an illness. The predisposition may never result in illness and the likelihood of illness developing even in someone with a predisposition depends more on stages in his life and environmental (extrinsic) factors.

The most likely times for mental illness to develop in any individual are puberty, pregnancy, the menopause, late middle age and retirement. As seen in Table 2.9 (page 30) mental illness is the commonest cause of days lost in women but only the fourth commonest in man.

(2) *Extrinsic* or environmental factors are even more complicated as each person continuously selects from his environment different features which he perceives. The more unsatisfactory and insecure the surroundings of anyone, the more likely it is that mental illness will develop but each person will react differently if placed in the same surroundings.

Once a mental illness has started, the longer the illness goes on, the more likely it is to be permanent, regardless of the detailed circumstances associated with its commencement. It is, therefore, important to try and diagnose even the very early signs of mental illness—in say a child—for early diagnosis will help treatment.

Many 'functional' disorders are due to bad social effects in childhood, or too rigid or ill-judged moral or cultural standards, or rejection by a parent. Many such problems are met with by social workers, health visitors and school nurses in their ordinary work. More and more arrangements are being made to introduce preventive psychiatry into child care services, and many authorities have introduced psychiatrists into the routine work of the child health clinic and in work in community homes with disturbed deprived children.

It is important to realize that it is impossible to protect any person from all mental or physical trauma in life—in fact, attempts to do this may very well encourage mental breakdown. It is, however, always possible to alter an environment in one way or another and this may help to avoid an impending illness.

The occupation and work which a person does has an important effect on his mental stability. Much illness can be averted by employment suitable for the person. Careful medical and psychological testing before people are placed in various occupations can help to avoid subsequent mental illness.

Training schemes, as described in Chapter 15, for mentally handicapped persons are invaluable in helping them to be rehabilitated. Great care must always be taken with the placement of children with severe emotional or behavioural disorders in industry when they leave school.

Finally, it is most important that sensible, true and balanced advice is always given. Health education programmes should always be alive to the dangers of wrong advice which may be handed down from parents and grandparents. Many needless fears can be caused in this way and these, in a person predisposed to mental illness, may be the spark which starts off an illness.

9
Health Education

This book describes some of the ways in which disease can be prevented or alleviated by widespread community services in both the health and social fields. But all these services can only succeed if they are widely accepted and used by the public. The process of persuading people to accept them and to avoid those things which will have an adverse effect is called **health education**.

Although most people are interested in factors which affect health, the final decisions of each individual are influenced by many different factors making up that person's total environment. The home, the school, the moral teaching, the prejudices and bias, the occupation, all can influence decisions.

Much sickness is the result of faulty personal or community habits including excessive eating and drinking or a lack of exercise or cigarette smoking. Most cases of cancer of the lung, chronic bronchitis and alcoholism come into this category and a small proportion of ischaemic heart disease attacks.

Because these factors are so varied, successful health education must influence the attitudes of individual people and, therefore, must permeate into the home, family life, school, work place and recreation. Health education, if it is to be successful, must therefore have access to as many people as possible—to parents, young children, adolescents, adults, elderly persons, teachers, employees, employers in all sections of the community.

It is most important to realize that *health education is not the sole responsibility of a professional health educator* but concerns doctors, health visitors, nurses, teachers and social workers. It is the aim of these to ensure that many members of the public also play a role in health education—parents, employers, trades union officials, youth leaders, church leaders, politicians, etc. In this way, the educating role becomes spread out and the end effects should be equally widespread throughout the community. By these means, ordinary people will be most likely to learn the best ways to maintain positive health.

Organization of health education

The Secretary of State for Social Services has overall responsibility for the policy and conduct and development of health education. Centrally many functions are delegated to the Health Education Council Ltd. Locally the District Health Authority through its District Medical Officer is responsible for health education. Local government still retains some health educational functions mainly in respect of the educational services and to a lesser extent in their environmental health and their social services.

Local

Health education is the responsibility of each District Health Authority under section 28 of the National Health Service Act, 1946. The District Medical Officer is locally in charge of the promotion of health education. Many health education problems are epidemiological and the most important causes of morbidity and mortality must be known before an effective local course of action can be planned to improve the health of that community. It is therefore important to measure local health problems carefully using various statistics (see Chapter 2).

Many different professionals play a vital part in this work:

(a) **Health education officers**. Just over half of all health authorities employ such staff. Many of these officers have had training in a nursing, health visiting or teaching field. Their main function is the organization and promotion of health education by:

(i) training staff to carry out group or individual health education

(ii) collecting and distributing suitable material and information

(iii) assessing and evaluating the impact of the health education undertaken.

(b) **Health visitors** (see Chapter 4) are probably more involved in detailed health education than any other health workers. Much of this work occurs when helping the young mother during her pregnancy or after her confinement by giving advice regarding the care of the baby. Any mother is very receptive to health education at such a time for she realizes that the health and proper development of her child rest mainly on the care she takes. She is, therefore, very anxious and keen to do all she can and usually listens carefully to the expert advice of the health visitor.

The health visitor is also very much concerned with giving health education advice to older children in school, to adolescents, to adults (especially those facing physical or mental handicaps) and also to the increasing number of elderly persons in the community.

The attachment of the health visitor to general practice increases her opportunities to promote health education.

(c) **General practitioners** have many opportunities for health education especially as the majority of patients have great faith in their doctor's advice. It is important that each doctor realizes the opportunities of carrying out health education at all times during his practice.

(d) **Nursing staff** at all times should also realize they have many chances to help people by educating them in the best ways to promote health and to avoid disease.

(e) **Teachers** also have a widespread influence on the lives of their pupils. School life always plays an important part in health education, as any success with children moulds the attitudes of future generations. If children learn how best to avoid disease and maintain good health at school, they are most likely to ensure their own children benefit in the same way.

(f) **Social workers** are also involved especially when dealing with children, physically and mentally handicapped persons and those of retirement age.

It will be understood from this list that *health education is a multi-disciplinary task* and that the rôle of the professional health education officer is mainly to help others to play a useful part.

National—The Health Education Council Ltd.

The national body set up to organize health education is the *Health Education Council Ltd.* This body has an annual budget of over a million pounds, most of which comes as a direct grant from the Department of Health and Social Security, the Welsh Office and the Department of Health and Social Services, Northern Ireland.

The main functions of the Health Education Council include:

1 To advise on priorities for health education.
2 To advise and carry out national or local campaigns in co-operation with health authorities or local authorities.
3 To produce information and publicity material and to publish articles of interest to those engaged in health education.
4 To sponsor and undertake research—this includes epidemiological and statistical research, cost benefit analysis and evaluation.
5 To act as the national centre of expertise in health education.
6 To encourage and promote training in health education work.
7 To cooperate with local education authorities in schools, colleges and polytechnics.
8 To maintain contact with and advise various national voluntary bodies engaged in specialized aspects of health education work.

Voluntary bodies and commercial organizations

Many different voluntary bodies are involved nationally in health education especially in the field of **accident prevention** e.g. the Royal Society for the Prevention of Accidents (RoSPA), and in cancer education. Commercial organizations mainly prepare visual aid material for use in health education—films, videotapes, filmstrips, slides. Some of these have both a self-advertising and health educational content. However, much of this commercial advertising is discreetly carried out and such films can be most useful.

Methods and techniques used in health education

Much skill is needed in successful health education for it is never sufficient just to tell people about a special subject. If possible, those being taught should be involved themselves and be motivated. This means successful health education must depend on first learning as much as possible about the audience. Discussion and argument are valuable and teaching sessions should never be too long. Visual aids of various kinds should be widely used as most people find it easier to learn more quickly in that way.

There are four main methods of health education:

(a) individual health education
(b) group health education
(c) mass media health education
(d) special campaigns.

(a) Individual health education

This is always the most effective because most people learn quickly this way and the results are more lasting. Personal discussions between patients and doctors, nurses and health visitors and simple demonstrations in the person's own home are most effective. Much individual health education can most naturally be carried out in connection with ordinary medical, nursing or social work in the course of day to day tasks. The **general practitioner** is usually in the ideal position to carry out effective personal education as the patient and family have complete faith in him, which is always an important factor in all teaching. While treating patients, the general practitioner should notice conditions within the home and, where necessary, give advice to improve them. In this way accidents will be reduced and diet and food hygiene improved.

Much of the most valuable health education which the **health visitor** carries out is effected while visiting the patient's home rather than at a clinic. Health education given in this way is more personal and effective. It is invariably very practical because advice is being given in the surroundings in which the patient must carry it out—in his or her own home and environment.

(b) Group health education

This occurs when small groups of people (six to eight) are taught together in child health clinics, schools or factories. Wherever possible, group discussions should be promoted so that everyone plays an active part. Talks should be short (10–15 minutes) and various visual aids should be used—film strips, colour slides, 16 mm films or video tapes.

Group health education can be particularly useful when the individual finds it difficult to follow the health advice being given as in the case of someone attempting to give up smoking or to lose weight. The group itself helps to support the individual in these instances.

(c) Mass media health education

In this technique, the subject is presented to the whole community by means of radio, television, posters and other methods designed to keep certain topics in the public eye.

Many different types of subject can be taught by this means—examples include the prevention of accidents, immunization, nutrition, the dangers of smoking and of sexually transmitted diseases. Much mass media health education is only effective if it is supported by other means, e.g., by individual and group discussions.

(d) Special health education campaigns

Examples of recent successful health education campaigns mounted by the Health Education Council include:

1 Smoking in pregnancy emphasizing the dangers that can be created for the unborn child
2 Alcoholism
3 Safe handling of medicines.

Local campaigns are also mounted from time to time to encourage a certain topic, e.g., immunization or accident prevention. Excellent results can be obtained in this way by using a '**community mobilization technique**' whereby volunteers are recruited to visit 15–20 homes to persuade the occupants to co-operate. Spectacular results have been obtained in this way as seen in the most successful mass X-ray campaigns held in Glasgow and Liverpool (see page 107).

It is important to realize that health education campaigns have two limitations:

1 all campaigns can be effective only for a short period of 3–4 weeks.

2   a very successful campaign may be followed by a dangerous lack of
    interest.

This is seen particularly in campaigns held to boost immunization.
Because of this feature, it is essential to combine the use of campaigns with
other methods of health education so that the improvements will be more
lasting.

Concentration on special problems

Occasionally it is necessary to concentrate health education on new
problems that are developing within a community to prevent them
becoming permanent. An example is *drug misuse* which is currently an
increasing menace. In tackling any such problem, there will always be two
main facets:

1   *primary prevention* to reduce the likelihood of more victims becoming
    involved;
2   *secondary prevention* to help those already misusing drugs and to
    prevent further deterioration of their condition.

In drug misuse one of the greatest difficulties to overcome is to build up
an effective communication system with those already taking drugs.
Special arrangements may have to be made and special workers or
volunteers have to be used.

Examples of health education

Most of the community health or social problems discussed in this book
can be influenced by health education. *Much prevention of disease and of
social problems depends on health education*, i.e., persuading people to act
early enough to prevent a disease starting or a social problem from
developing. Health education is important at all ages, but especially in
childhood, pregnancy and early motherhood and in old age.
    The list of health education topics is a long one and to avoid
duplication, the reader is referred to the appropriate chapter. The topics
include:

1   Ante-natal care (Chapter 3)
2   All aspects of child health care (Chapter 4)
3   Child care (Chapter 13)
4   Prevention of disease by immunization (Chapter 6)
5   Accident prevention in children (Chapter 4) and in old age (Chap-
    ter 16)
6   Nutrition (Chapter 8)

7   Prevention of communicable disease (Chapter 7)
8   Smoking (Chapter 8)
9   Sexually transmitted diseases (Chapter 7)
10 Cancer education (Chapter 8)
11 Dental care (Chapter 5)
12 Atmospheric pollution and other environmental health problems (Chapter 11).

10
International Disease Control

The control of international health has become increasingly important in a world in which the rate of travel from one country to another is becoming progressively faster.

The international controlling body for health in the world is the World Health Organization (WHO) which was set up from the work of an expert committee of the Economic and Social Council of the United Nations in 1946.

By 1981, there were 155 member states in WHO including all the major powers in the world.

The headquarters of WHO is at Geneva but there are 6 regions:

Africa with headquarters at Brazzaville
Americas with headquarters at Washington D.C.
East Mediterranean with headquarters at Alexandria, Egypt.
Europe with headquarters at Copenhagen
S. E. Asia with headquarters at New Delhi
West Pacific with headquarters at Manila, Phillipines.

Each region has its own Regional Advisory Committee on medical research but there is a single co-ordinating Global Advisory Committee.

Although WHO is concerned with all problems of health, it has always paid particular attention to the value of preventive medicine and has always played an important rôle in stimulating and assisting in developing the preventive medical services of the under-developed countries.

The principle that has been constantly followed by WHO is that 'health is now a world responsibility . . . for health, like peace, is one and indivisible'.

At present the six regions are concentrating upon different health topics—Africa upon developing and training health aids, Americas on an expanded programme of immunization, Eastern Mediterranean upon tapping human resources and upon the imbalance of health workers there, Europe upon food safety, South East Asia upon developing different forms of health care and Western Pacific upon developing community participation to encourage better health education and understanding.

A WHO Executive Board meets twice a year in Geneva and a World Health Assembly meets annually. Examples of successful co-operation among member states included the recent eradication of smallpox from the world. In 1978 the World Health Assembly accepted as a new universal aim the theme 'Health for all by Year 2000'.

An excellent popular health journal called *World Health* is published monthly as well as many technical and scientific papers.

Reporting service run by the World Health Organization on the world-wide incidence of serious infectious disease

The WHO publishes weekly a bulletin on the world-wide incidence of serious infectious diseases and particularly on:

Plague	Cholera
Yellow Fever	Typhus
	Relapsing fever

This bulletin contains exact details of numbers of such cases and the cities and ports in which they have occurred throughout the world. It also records brief details of other unusually large epidemics (such as influenza) which may be occurring in different parts of the world. It notes any changes made locally by a country in its immunization or vaccination requirements so that those advising travellers are kept informed.

These bulletins are invaluable as a reliable up-to-date record of the incidence of serious infection and are of the utmost importance to medical officers at all large ports and airports.

A daily epidemiological radio-telegraphic bulletin is broadcast by the World Health Organization from:

Geneva	Keelung
Saigon	Manila

and once or twice a week broadcasts from

Tokyo	Karachi
Hongkong	Madras
Singapore	Mauritius.

Port and airport health control

Present methods of health clearance at ports include an arrangement whereby masters of ships must report by radio in advance of their arrival the occurrence of any illness in terms of signs and symptoms rather than specific diseases. Where necessary a doctor visits and, in addition, a random sample of ships is subjected to inspection. A similar system operates satisfactorily at airports.

Control of imported foods likely to cause disease

Additional preventive medical work undertaken by the port health staff includes the examination of all imports of foodstuffs into this country to make certain that no unsound or diseased food stuffs are imported, which might later lead to disease. Stringent regulations are laid down concerning food imports. All meat, for instance, that is imported must be in a recognizable form and must bear *the official certificate* of the country of origin, stating that it has been properly inspected. In addition, food inspectors carefully examine the meat for signs of disease which, if found, results in the condemnation of that meat.

All tinned products are also tested to make certain that tins are sound. A small proportion are further examined by a bacteriologist to ensure that the tins have been properly processed and the contents sterilized.

Egg products that are imported are also carefully sampled and examined. In recent years investigations and sampling have shown that some egg imports were infected with salmonella bacteria which cause food poisoning. Much research work finally developed a satisfactory heat treatment process whereby such products can be rendered completely safe for human consumption without altering the nature of the egg albumen.

Desiccated coconut was another imported foodstuff shown to be infected with salmonella bacteria. These imports came from Sri Lanka and, as a result of the findings, the government of Sri Linka has improved greatly the standard of production.

Further preventive work carried out by WHO

The main concern of WHO is to induce self help in countries by sending small teams of experts to the under-developed countries to study their methods and suggest ways in which the preventive health services can be improved. This has been done very successfully in many places and, as a result of the improvements introduced, the infant mortality of some of the worst under-developed countries has already been dramatically reduced.

Communicable disease control

Some of the most successful preventive medical work of the World Health Organization has been in the control of widespread communicable diseases in many countries.

Malaria

The control of malaria has been one of the major aims of WHO since its formation.

This work has been so successful that the annual number of malaria deaths has dropped significantly. There are however still approximately 1200 million people in the world who are at risk of contracting malaria and at present the numbers are rising. However indigenous malaria has already been completely eradicated from much of the world (i.e. the total North American continent and Mexico). All countries still see imported cases. In England and Wales in 1981, 1268 cases were recorded but the vast majority of these occurred in immigrants and their children. This figure has risen dramatically in the last six years (595 cases in 1975) but the rate of increases has now dropped.

The work of WHO in malaria control has always been concentrated:

(a) upon improving treatment facilities to reduce the effect of the attack and the chances of subsequent infection to others

(b) upon preventive measures which are specially planned

(i) to improve the environmental factors which, if faulty, encourage mosquito multiplication and aid the spread of malaria. These include the drainage of swamps, ditches and other stagnant water, and widespread spraying with insecticide. To assist in this work, a number of expert sanitary engineers are employed by WHO to visit countries and give advice:

(ii) to introduce medical preventive measures whereby populations at special risk receive drugs regularly as a prophylactic.

In addition, many research studies in the problems of malaria are encouraged and financed by WHO including:

1   Susceptibility of mosquitoes to new insecticides;
2   Researches using medicated salt to give populations prophylactic drugs;
3   Studies in drug resistance;
4   Studies on new anti-malarial drugs.

Cholera

WHO has been very active in planning programmes for the prevention of cholera especially in India and the East. During the past decade, the *El Tor* cholera vibrio has almost completely replaced the classic strain.

In 1971 there was a threat of a cholera pandemic when over 171 000 cases were traced in 38 countries. Since then numbers have fallen but the international surveillance of cholera has been one of the major tasks of WHO. It constantly receives, consolidates and disseminates epidemiological information about cholera incidence in its weekly bulletins. As many of the countries at greatest risk of cholera epidemics have limited health resources, much of the work of WHO has been to help research into finding suitable methods for cholera surveillance. Vaccination results against this type of cholera have been disappointing.

Tuberculosis

Tuberculosis has been the target for many preventive medical campaigns launched by the WHO. Work has included widespread immunization campaigns using BCG vaccine as well as the detailed planning of many national programmes for the proper treatment and control of this disease.

A widespread training programme for medical and nursing personnel has been arranged so that self help in the fight against tuberculosis can be encouraged in all countries.

The cost of certain anti-tuberculosis drugs such as PAS has been too prohibitive for some developing countries and research has been promoted by the World Health Organization to find cheaper alternative drugs.

One of the great problems in the eradication of tuberculosis which the World Health Organization has found, has been the *indifference of patients in the self-administration of anti-tuberculosis drugs.*

WHO has supported research into tuberculosis in:

(a) developing international quality control of BCG vaccine

(b) development of cheap and effective combination of drugs for treating the disease

(c) studies of drug resistance

(d) investigations into jet methods of injection of vaccines.

Sexually transmitted diseases

Many researches into the level of sexually transmitted diseases in many under-developed countries have been carried out by the World Health Organization.

At the World Health Assembly held in 1975 a resolution was passed requesting all Governments to consider the need;

1 to make optimal use of existing services and health structures to strengthen the control of sexually transmitted diseases,
2 to encourage the appropriate training, in this field, of medical personnel and other workers at all levels and the further training of existing personnel,
3 to promote information and health education to all concerned in order to develop the sense of responsibility and respect for the integrity of all human beings.

Leprosy

The World Health Organization has been very active in developing services for the recognition and early treatment of leprosy.

In high endemic areas, special emphasis has been given to surveys of schoolchildren. In one recent survey in Burma, the rate of leprosy in schoolchildren was found to be 36 per thousand. Early treatment of such cases prevents these children becoming open cases and developing disabilities, and will also reduce the contagiousness of the disease.

Special World Health Organization advisory teams are constantly visiting affected countries to carry out surveys, give advice on anti-leprosy programmes and on the training of the countries' own medical workers.

The World Health Organization has also continued to support and carry out research into the transmission of human leprosy, chemotherapeutic methods of treatment and the epidemiology of leprosy.

Trachoma

This disease of the eye which so often leads to blindness has been one of the constant medical problems of many tropical countries. WHO has continuously helped in campaigns designed to prevent this disease. Widespread help has been given by the Organization in awarding fellowships for work on trachoma research.

Special teaching courses have been constantly arranged for ophthalmologists, in laboratory, clinical and epidemiological techniques.

Consultant services are also provided to help countries develop their own trachoma control services.

Rabies

The WHO is playing an increasing rôle in providing up-to-date information on the spread of rabies in wild animals especially in Europe.

General work of WHO

In addition, the WHO has undertaken much international preventive work connected with the control of yaws, the parasitic diseases including bilharziasis, trypanosomiasis, filarial infections, leishmaniasis and mycotic diseases.

The World Health Organization is also responsible for recommending changes in *international quarantine*.

Other preventive and research work assisted or supported by WHO includes:

1 Many types of vaccine trials
2 Promotion of maternity and child health services
3 Research into causation of accidents
4 Research into mental health
5 Studies in environmental health
6 Research into cardiovascular diseases
7 Studies into social and occupational health
8 Research into human genetics
9 Nutritional studies
10 Promotion of dental health
11 Health education
12 Development of nursing services
13 Prevention of radiation hazards
14 Development of health laboratory services
15 Drug addiction studies
16 Standardization of pharmaceutical drugs and products

The World Health Organization also arranges for many travelling medical and nursing fellowships so that there is a high level of co-ordination in world health services.

11
Environmental Health Control

Many of the everyday factors within our lives can have a marked effect upon our health. These include the area and house we live in, the atmosphere we breathe, the food we eat and the water we drink. Usually in a civilized well-developed country, most of these factors are well controlled and their effect upon health is often forgotten. In primitive communities, however, the connection between environment and health is more obvious as there is often much communicable disease spread in this way.

In this chapter, *environmental* health problems are considered to show what effect on health environmental defects can produce.

Housing and town planning

The house a person lives in has an important influence upon that individual's life and well-being. It also has a significant effect upon health.

A satisfactory house must reach certain physical standards, such as being free from dampness, being well lighted and ventilated, having a proper water system including hot water system and bath, an adequate internal water closet, sinks and proper drainage system, adequate means for preparing, storing and cooking food. These physical standards are invariably found in modern houses, but many of the older houses especially in industrial areas lack some of them.

The house must also be suitable for the family living there, and this means that not only must it be large enough, but it should be sited in an attractive way not being too close to other houses, and form an integral part of a group of houses or area.

No family living in an inadequate house will be able to enjoy life completely. But nor will all the families of a large area be able to live properly unless all the necessary community services—shops, churches, schools, doctors' houses, health centres and hospitals, community centres, cinemas, etc., are present. In communities such as a country town which has developed over many years—often centuries—all such facilities will usually be present for they have been added to the community gradually.

It is in the area which has developed quickly in which so many of these facilities are missing. Examples include:

(a) 'Slum' areas in industrial towns which were built in the last century when the absence of transport led factory owners to crowd together too many houses in small areas. With the bad planning of these houses and their deterioration, they now provide overcrowded, unpleasant, damp and unhealthy homes.

(b) many new housing estates contain sound houses but all too often the necessary community facilities are absent. So, hundreds of houses may be built without all the essential community services, such as shops, being provided.

It is now known that it is best to plan a whole neighbourhood unit in all urban development. Since 1948, new towns and housing areas have always attempted to follow the neighbourhood unit plan. Developments should not be too large, and a neighbourhood unit for about 10 000 persons is considered ideal. Within such a development not only should the necessary houses be built but essential services such as shops, schools, churches, community centres, library, police station, clinics, health centres etc. should be provided.

Effects of bad housing on health

Although slum clearance—the demolition of unsuitable houses—has been going on since the 1920s, there still remain many poor houses in the large cities and industrial towns. What effect does such poor housing have upon the health of those living in it?

It is not difficult to demonstrate that the health of people living in slum areas is inferior to those living in good ones. There is a greater amount of communicable disease present, and when the children develop the usual childhood diseases, there is a higher incidence of complications. Overcrowding which is always present in slums leads to greater ease of infection of the air-borne diseases and the best example is pulmonary tuberculosis. This disease is commoner in the slum population. Acute rheumatic fever is also mainly seen today in children from slum areas.

The effect of the poor housing is often to make the individual *more liable* to disease than actually to produce disease. Many a patient living in bad housing who develops tuberculosis, feels the bad house has caused the disease. This, of course, is not so, for the disease has been caused by an attack on the lung by the tubercle bacillus. But the poor housing and living conditions have made the accident of infection more likely.

The majority of poor houses are damp—either from defective roofs or gutters allowing rain water to enter the house, or by rising dampness percolating upwards from the ground, due to the absence of a damp-proof course. Damp living conditions lead to an exacerbation of various *rheumatic problems* so commonly found later in life, a *higher child mortality*, and a greater incidence of serious chest conditions such as *acute bronchitis*. Such conditions also aggravate *chronic bronchitis* in the elderly.

Dampness always has a most depressing effect on the occupants of the home who see their efforts at redecoration ruined and leads to much unhappiness and aggravation of minor mental and emotional disorders.

The overcrowding effect of poor housing has a stultifying effect upon the proper development of the family. It is obvious that no family can hope to reach its full potential in such conditions—children cannot walk properly and their school development suffers—adults give up because the effort to overcome the difficulties becomes too great. The extra strain of looking after a mentally handicapped child in such conditions is tremendous and is often so difficult that the child has to be admitted to hospital although he could have stayed happily at home if only the house had been more suitable.

Poor housing cannot be said to be a cause of mental illness but it certainly is a contributory factor and has a very bad and often disastrous effect on the mentally ill patient living there. Even after the acute state of the mental illness has passed, unsatisfactory home conditions can retard recovery.

The *level of accidents* both in children and old persons is much higher in those living in poor houses. This is due to bad lighting and steep unsuitable stairs which predispose to falling accidents. Overcrowding also is associated with an increased number of scalds and burns.

Poor housing conditions not only predispose the individual to attacks of some diseases but may also be a most important factor in the *correct management of illness*. A patient with angina of effort or a chronic cardiac condition must be able to avoid stairs. In a modern house, it is usually possible to arrange this by turning a downstairs room into a temporary bedroom and this works quite well, especially if there is a downstairs lavatory. But in the slum house, this would be impossible and the management of such a case is made difficult. Either the patient would have to climb steep stairs or stay permanently upstairs; there is also the complication that in the slum house there is not usually an inside lavatory.

The management of various forms of malignant disease is made very difficult in slum houses. A case with a colostomy, for instance, will produce many extra problems in the absence of a bathroom, internal lavatory and proper washing facilities.

Local authorities realize the importance of doing all they can to provide good houses. It is usual for the housing authority to give *special priority for urgent housing for really important medical reasons* so that the effect of poor housing on health can be minimized. Much tuberculosis infection is prevented in this way by the rapid rehousing of a patient's family if they are living in an overcrowded slum house.

Methods of dealing with unsatisfactory houses

Unsatisfactory houses can be dealt with in a number of ways:

(a) slight defects can be put right by using s. 93 of the Public Health Act 1936 and serving an abatement notice on the owner.

(b) individual unfit houses can be demolished or repaired (s. 16–17 Housing Act 1957).

(c) houses or parts of houses may be closed.

(d) large Clearance Areas can be defined under s. 42 Housing Act 1957. This is the usual method used for large scale slum clearance. The Department of the Environment holds a local inquiry where the council has to provide public evidence of unfitness of houses and where owners can bring their own evidence.

(e) houses in multiple occupation can be controlled (Part II Housing Act 1961).

(f) special measures can be used to improve houses.

All these methods are used by the environmental health inspectors who are responsible for this work.

Atmospheric pollution and health

Although atmospheric pollution has improved markedly in the last few years, many large cities and towns, especially those in industrial areas, have their atmosphere constantly polluted by smoke and other fumes in the air. It is known that the health of the people living in such areas is affected by this atmospheric contamination.

Atmospheric pollution is probably a small factor in the production of lung cancer, for it is known that the level of lung cancer is higher in industrial areas than in country areas. It is a minor problem compared with cigarette smoking, but is a factor.

However, the most serious danger to health occurs in those unfortunate people who have some degree of *chronic bronchitis*. Many of these are elderly and their respiratory and cardiac function is impaired. The climate of this country with its damp misty winter days always tends to make such patients worse but really serious medical problems arise when atmospheric pollution in the form of a smoky fog (smog) occurs. To such patients even minor pollution increases their symptoms while a major fog, lasting a few days, often brings them very near complete collapse. For instance, in the historic smog of London in December 1952, it is estimated that just under 4000 patients with chronic bronchitis died. The inhalation of smoky particles and/or sulphur gases commonly present in industrial areas both play a part in aggravating the chronic bronchitic's condition.

Living in an atmosphere that is always dirty has a most depressing effect upon people and adds greatly to their daily problems. Since the Clean Air Act came into force in 1956, local authorities have progressed towards the ideal of clearing the atmosphere of all pollution. It was hoped to achieve this by:

(a) preventing the building of any new factory plant unless its means of producing heat or power are completely smokeless. *Prior approval* of all such plans must be given by local authorities before any building construction can start;

(b) introducing *smoke control areas* in which it is an offence to produce any smoke at all or to burn ordinary coal. Before any part of a town can be made such an area, all the houses must have cooking and heating methods which are smokeless. This may mean replacing old grates with modern ones capable of burning smokeless fuel. A more satisfactory method is to change to other forms of power such as oil, gas or electricity. To help the householder to meet the cost of these conversions, 70 per cent of the cost is paid by a grant from the local authority who in turn get 40 per cent from the central government. This means the householder pays 30 per cent of the cost. This grant is only given for conversions necessary to comply with the introduction of a new smoke control area.

Already in most industrial towns where smoke control areas have been widely introduced, there is a noticeable improvement in times of mist and fog. Unfortunately due to the financial recession, very few new smoke control areas have been introduced recently.

Food control

Many diseases that affect animals can also attack man. The prevention of such illnesses depends on the care and control of food production and on the various inspections taking place to avoid contaminated food ever being eaten by man.

Food inspection at ports

As much of our food is imported from abroad, a very careful inspection is made of all food arriving at the port of importation. Each consignment is inspected and sampled and can be imported only if the *port health staff* are satisfied as to its high standard.

All meat imported has to have a special certificate of purity from the country of origin and, in addition, is carefully examined by *meat inspectors*. If any disease is found, the complete carcase is given a very careful further examination. If the disease is only local, and the diseased portion can be completely removed, this is done. But, if the disease is widespread, the whole carcase is condemned and either has to be re-exported or destroyed, or stained and sent for animal foodstuff after complete sterilization. Certain meats are *prohibited meats* and cannot be imported, including:

(a) scrap meat which cannot be identified

(b) meat comprising parts of the wall of the thorax or abdomen from which any part of pleura or peritoneum has been detached

(c) meat, except mutton and lamb, from which a lymphatic gland has been taken out

(d) the head of an animal without a submaxillary gland.

Tinned goods are sampled and examined and a small sample is sent to a bacteriologist for a full and complete bacteriological examination to check on the sterility of the product. If the results are unsatisfactory, the whole consignment can be condemned and not allowed to be imported.

All types of foodstuffs are examined in the same careful way.

With many new independent countries developing, careful inspection and sampling of all imported foodstuffs is even more important than usual for, in the process of independence, there may be a temporary lowering of standards of cleanliness in food control. Sampling at the port is the great safeguard to ensure that no contaminated food can enter this country.

Meat inspection

Continuous meat inspection is undertaken on all meat produced and eaten in this country.

Meat is examined by specially trained inspectors immediately after slaughter in the abbatoir. A systematic, careful inspection is made of all carcases: if any disease is found, it is dealt with in the same way as already described in port meat inspection.

Tuberculosis was a disease which, forty years ago, was common in cattle in this country. Today it is very rarely seen, but it is still important to take steps to avoid meat infected with tuberculosis from ever coming into a kitchen, for if this occurs, infection is very likely, as working surfaces, such as tables, will soon become contaminated. The pathogenic bacteria in the meat might be destroyed by heat in the cooking, but other foodstuffs would rapidly be infected via the contaminated working surfaces. The Aberdeen typhoid epidemic of 1964 was probably spread in this way—from a contaminated counter in a cooked meat department of a supermarket.

For this reason, contaminated meat is only allowed to be used for animal foodstuffs provided it is sterilized and thoroughly stained with a dye to make such meat easily recognizable.

Other diseases commonly found in animal carcases include various animal parasites and tapeworms such as *Taenia solium, Trichinella spiralis,* hydatid cysts.

There are also a number of infectious conditions in animals which lead to the condemnation of the meat including various forms of *salmonellosis, septicaemia, anthrax, pyaemia* and *actinomycosis.*

Prevention of disease by control of milk supplies

Milk is a very important and essential part of our food supplies and forms the basis of all infant feeding. Milk supplies have always been particularly liable to lead to the spread of infectious disease because:

(a) the cow may suffer from two diseases which can be passed on to man via her milk—*tuberculosis* and *brucellosis*

(b) milk supplies may be contaminated in the process of collecting and distributing milk. In the past, before modern clean methods of milk distribution were perfected, epidemics traced to such causes included *typhoid, paratyphoid, diphtheria, scarlet fever* and other *streptococcal* infections, *food poisoning, dysentery, gastroenteritis* and *brucellosis*.

The prevention of milk infection in this country is now complete and it is extremely rare for infection of any kind to be traced to milk which has been heat treated or pasteurized and then only after very gross carelessness. It is, however, only relatively recently that such a satisfactory state has existed, for forty years ago much infectious disease was caused by milk.

The improvement has resulted from:

(a) a nationwide campaign by the Ministry of Agriculture, Fisheries and Food to eradicate tuberculosis from all dairy herds. This scheme, started modestly in the late 1930s, has rapidly been extended to include the majority of the country. This campaign, which was introduced with financial bonuses to encourage the farmer to keep a tuberculin free herd, has been so successful that today there is hardly any tuberculosis among cows.

The inspection of farms and equipment to ensure that good standards are maintained throughout the country, is undertaken by officials of the Ministry of Agriculture, Fisheries and Food.

(b) the large scale pasteurization of milk supplies. *Pasteurization of milk* means the subjection of the milk to heat treatment for a specified time so that any live pathogenic or disease-producing bacteria are killed. The usual process of pasteurization is the *High Temperature Short Time process* in which milk is retained at a temperature of not less than 71.5°C (161°F) for 15 seconds and then immediately cooled to a temperature of not more than 10°C (50°F).

Another but less popular method of pasteurization is by the *Holder* process in which the milk is maintained in a vat at a temperature of not less than 62.8°C (145°F) and not more than 65.5°C (150°F) for at least half an hour and then immediately cooled to a temperature of not more than 10°C (50°F). Both processes kill all pathogenic bacteria and so render the milk safe. No important food value is lost by pasteurization although the fat emulsion may be slightly affected and the cream does not rise as readily.

Immediately after pasteurization, the milk is bottled by machine and sealed so that no further chance of contamination can occur. In this way, the milk is delivered to the householder completely safe and free from infection.

Before the introduction of these safeguards, many children and young persons developed attacks of tuberculous cervical adenitis and tuberculous peritonitis as well as tuberculous infection of the bones and joints, and meningitis. Raw milk has also recently been shown to be the cause of a number of salmonella food poisoning outbreaks. Pasteurization is the only way to prevent such communicable diseases.

Sterilized milk is milk which has been filtered and homogenized and then maintained at a temperature of not less than 100°C (212°F) for such a period as to comply with the turbidity test. In practice the milk after filtering and homogenizing is poured into bottles and heated to 108°C (228°F) for 10–12 minutes.

Ultra-heat-treated (UHT) milk has been retained at a temperature of not less than 132°C (270°F) for a period of not less than one second, and then is immediately placed in sterile containers in which it is supplied to the consumer.

As a further precaution, any person working in a dairy shop who develops a communicable disease must notify the local 'proper officer' who is generally the District Medical Officer or another specially designated community physician. The 'proper officer' can prohibit the sale of milk if it is likely to cause disease, until it has been heat-treated.

The 'proper officer' can also prohibit any person who is an open infectious case of tuberculosis from working in a dairy or milking cows on a farm.

There is no doubt that the widespread powers in this country to prevent disease from being spread by milk have been most successful. Today pasteurized milk in this country is a completely safe and reliable food supply and is completely free from possible pathogenic bacteria such as brucellosis, tuberculosis or salmonellosis.

Sampling to prevent adulteration of milk and food supplies

The possible adulteration of food supplies is very carefully guarded against by the continuous sampling of all foodstuffs. It is important that the public must be able to rely on any food they buy being unadulterated. At the beginning of the century, there was widespread adulteration of food in this country and this led to disease due both to dangerous additives to food and the lowering of nutritional value of some foods which were diluted in this way.

The adding of water to milk is fortunately easily detected by a test on the freezing point of milk—the *adulterated milk has a higher freezing point*. Sampling of milk supplies goes on all the time and very heavy penalties are given to the rare offenders. The dilution of milk by adding water is not only grossly dishonest but as milk is used for the basis of infant feeding, could lead to undernutrition in babies.

Only very limited preservatives are allowed to be added to certain foods. It is illegal to add preservatives to the majority of foods including all milk products. This is because preservatives could mask staleness of food and encourage incorrect food storage which would make food poisoning attacks more likely. Examples of foods in which limited preservatives may be added are sausages, jams, and pickles.

Environmental health inspectors carry out sampling which, of course, is always without warning, on shops and stores selling food and drugs and drink. Samples are tested for purity and for any evidence of adulteration. This constant vigilance has resulted in a very high standard being maintained in all food products, and cases of adulteration are very rare.

Special precautions for special foodstuffs

Certain foodstuffs are particularly liable to contamination which may result in disease in man, and special precautions are necessary to avoid this. Good examples of such foods are shell-fish and ice cream.

Shell-fish

Many shell-fish are eaten raw. For this reason, special precautions must be taken to ensure that shell-fish do not become contaminated with pathogenic bacteria. Unfortunately shell-fish often contain *typhoid* and *paratyphoid bacilli* if they have been collected from a sea-shore or sea which is grossly contaminated with sewage. A number of outbreaks of typhoid fever have been caused in this way.

Many parts of our sea-shore are polluted, as crude sewage is often emptied into river mouths.

Special regulations are enforced preventing the collection of shell-fish from dangerously polluted beaches. Shell-fish can be purified by immersion in specially prepared tanks for two to three weeks, and this is carried out commercially in certain places to make certain that no danger of spreading typhoid exists.

Ice cream

Ice cream is particularly liable to spread infection because, although bacteria will not multiply at the low temperatures necessary for ice cream, the bacteria present in ice cream will be preserved at such temperatures. This means that a disease like *typhoid fever* which can easily be spread by a tiny infecting dose could be spread widely by ice cream which has become contaminated with typhoid bacilli. This is exactly what happened in the Aberystwyth ice cream typhoid outbreak in 1945 when over 100 cases of typhoid occurred.

To prevent any possible recurrence, *all ice cream must, by law, now be pasteurized* and then cooled and left at a temperature not above 9.3°C (45°F) until frozen. This compulsory pasteurization has prevented the danger of further epidemics of typhoid.

Special preventive measures relating to food handlers

Under Food Hygiene (General) Regulations 1970 special precautions must be taken by all food handlers in shops and stalls to avoid spreading disease. These include:

(a) All steps must be taken to avoid food becoming contaminated—food must be covered and protected from flies and contact with the public.

(b) No open food—that is food not in a tin or jar—must be placed lower than 18 inches (45 cm) from the ground.

(c) Anybody handling food must keep his person and clothes clean.

(d) Any open cut or abrasion must be covered by a waterproof dressing. This is to avoid staphylococcal lesions in whitlows, boils, etc., from contaminating food and causing a food poisoning.

(e) All food handlers must refrain from spitting and smoking.

(f) All wrapping paper must be clean—newspapers are not allowed except for uncooked vegetables.

(g) Any food handler who becomes aware that he is suffering from *typhoid* or *paratyphoid fever, salmonella* infection, *dysentery* or *staphylococcal* infection, must notify the 'proper officer'—the District Medical Officer or another specially designated community physician.

In addition, there are widespread regulations about food premises all designed to reduce the chance of infection. These include regulations about the provisions of washing facilities with hot and cold water, working surfaces to prevent accumulation of bacteria in cracks on unsuitable types of surfaces. Also standards are laid down for the construction of premises and the temperature at which foods may be stored.

Further regulations concern many aspects of the transport and handling of foodstuffs. All are designed to prevent the spread of disease.

Control of water supplies

In this country, the control of water supplies, their purification and cleanliness has been so reliable that one hardly considers that this is an important health safeguard. The disastrous epidemic of typhoid in Zermatt, in Switzerland, in 1963 reminds one of the dangers which face any population which ignores stringent high safety standards.

There are two bacterial diseases spread by water—*typhoid fever* and *cholera*. Cholera is a disease seen mainly in the East which can spread because of grossly inadequate water and sewage systems. Its epidemic spread today in this country is virtually impossible.

But typhoid fever could quite easily be spread by water unless constant care is taken to ensure that the purification of water is complete. This entails:

(a) storage of water in reservoirs;
(b) filtration of water;
(c) sterilization of water using chlorine to make certain that any bacteria not removed by filtration are killed.

In addition, great care is always needed to make certain that no employee in a water works contaminates the supply. In particular, *it is essential to make certain that no typhoid carriers are ever employed in a water works.* Careful medical tests including agglutination blood tests are carried out on all such employees to reduce the chance of a carrier not being detected among the staff of the water works. The last serious water-borne outbreak of typhoid fever in this country was in Croydon in 1937 when 290 cases of typhoid fever occurred. It was caused by a urinary carrier contaminating the water supply while he assisted in work on a deep well forming part of Croydon's water supply.

Very high standards are maintained in the water supplies in this country and further large scale outbreaks of water-borne typhoid are most unlikely to occur. The most vulnerable supplies are probably some country ones especially during the crowded holiday months of July and August. Constant sampling of all water supplies, is an extra safeguard for such sampling will immediately show if the purity of the water supply has suddenly deteriorated.

The freedom of infection from water supplies in this country is no guide to the hazards of many foreign countries. *Many cases of typhoid occur each year in travellers from the Indian sub-continent, Italy, Spain and North Africa* especially when these visitors have stayed in remote country areas or on camping holidays. If such a holiday is planned, it is essential either:

(i) to *sterilize all water* with a simple camp sterilization outfit; or

(ii) to be *protected with a course of TAB inoculation* before starting. This protects against typhoid fever and paratyphoid fever (see page 93).

Fluoridation of water supplies

It is known that the variation in dental caries found in different areas is connected with the content of natural fluoride in the water consumed by the people of that area (see page 136).

In localities where the natural fluoride content of the water supply is low, fluoride can be added to the water supply to bring the level to about one part of fluoride per million parts of water. This has been done in many parts of the world and has always been followed by a substantial reduction in the amount of dental caries in the children in that area. After pilot trials, the Department of Health and Social Security has advised that all water supplies should have fluoride added to them where the natural supply of fluoride is deficient. It is known that if this is done, there should be a reduction of at least 60 per cent in the dental caries. A number of areas (about 7 per cent of England and Wales) have already introduced artificial fluoridation. Unfortunately ill-informed persons have campaigned very forcibly against fluoridation on the grounds that it is 'mass medication' and an intrusion into their individual liberty.

This attitude is very difficult to understand when it is realized that chlorine is added to all water supplies for safety. There is ample evidence that fluoridation would be a most valuable preventive medical factor and would undoubtedly result in far less pain and suffering in children from dental caries. It is to be hoped that this public reaction will not be allowed to interfere with what is a most valuable preventive dental service.

12
Structure of the Social Services

The 'social services' in the United Kingdom cover many different types of services but mainly fall into three well-defined groups:

1 Social services provided by *local authority social services departments* which include a wide range of statutory, domiciliary and residential services for children, physically disabled, mentally disabled, homeless and elderly people. Since 1974, the hospital social work services are also provided by local authorities although such work is entirely undertaken within a hospital setting.

These types of social services are described in Chapters 13 to 16, each chapter dealing with one of the client groups listed above. Centrally these services are the responsibility of the Secretary of State for Social Services and the Department of Health and Social Security.

2 The *probation and aftercare service* which is attached to the courts and works mainly with adult offenders who, as part of their sentence, are placed on probation. In addition, much of the aftercare work for discharged prisoners is undertaken by this service. Note that much of the court aftercare work of juvenile offenders (delinquent children) is carried out by local authority social services (see Chapter 13).

The probation service is quite separate from the local authority social services and, like the Prison Service, is centrally the responsibility of the Home Secretary and the Home Office.

3 *Voluntary Bodies.* There are many well established voluntary bodies providing social services of all kinds both on a national and local basis. They include specialist bodies working with children, such as NSPCC, Barnardos, National Children's Homes, the Family Welfare Association, and groups dealing with the elderly, such as Age Concern. The Women's Royal Voluntary Service covers a wide range of voluntary help while the Family Service Units provide assistance to problem families. There are many specialist voluntary bodies working in the field of the disabled including the Central Council for the Disabled and the British Council for the Rehabilitation of the Disabled. Locally Councils of Social Service and Rural Community Councils undertake a co-ordinating rôle in respect of many small voluntary bodies or local branches of the large national bodies.

Many of these voluntary bodies are providing services which could also be undertaken by Social Service Departments and it is therefore essential that very close working arrangements are made. In many instances, much of the finance necessary for their function is provided by the Social Services Committee of the Local Authority.

Nationally the government department which is mainly responsible for voluntary bodies is the Department of Health and Social Security; in some instances this department encourages voluntary work in the social services by providing small grants to voluntary bodies especially in respect of experimental schemes. Examples of such grants recently made include financial help to reduce and prevent alcoholism.

A further example of voluntary work in the social services is the Citizens' Advice Bureaux. These were first developed in the 1939–45 war to help various queries about rationing, missing relatives, etc. Their rôle has been widened recently to include consumer protection, the provision of legal advice and the explanation of various pension rights. They are particularly valuable in helping families who may be unwilling to seek help from statutory services (such as a Social Service Department) because they may feel aggrieved for some reason—they may have been evicted for rent arrears or generally are resentful of the way they have been treated in the past by local authorities and other statutory services. For this reason many local authority Social Services Committees give financial grants to the Citizens' Advice Bureaux to enable them to help clients who otherwise would be unlikely to seek help. Centrally there is a National Association of Citizens' Advice Bureaux linked to local bureaux by a regional committee.

Local authority social services

Social services for children, physically disabled, mentally disabled, homeless and elderly people are provided by large–local authorities—by the metropolitan districts in the large conurbations or by the London boroughs in London, and by the county councils in the rest of England and Wales (see Figure 12.2, page 179).

Central Government Control of Local Authority Social Services

The main government department in England which is concerned with the administration of local authority social services is the Department of Health and Social Security. The Minister in charge is the Secretary of State for Social Services, a member of the Cabinet, and who is also responsible for both the health services (see page 1) and for social security (see Chapter 18), the system which supports those in need of financial help because of illness, disablement or old age.

The reason for having the same senior minister (Secretary of State for Social Services) and the same government department (Department of Health and Social Security) responsible for social services, health services and social security, is that all three are very closely related. Most families will need all three from time to time for social services provide the main supporting services in the community for children, the disabled (physically and mentally handicapped and mentally ill), the homeless and the aged. Social security provides various allowances or pensions for the family—child benefit, widows' pensions, sickness benefit claims, old age pensions and family income supplement (see Chapter 18). Medical services for the family are, of course, provided by the health services (see Chapter 1).

The rôle of the Department of Health and Social Security in social services is similar to that described for the health services (see pages 2–4), for the Department is primarily concerned in assisting the development of social services in three main ways:

(a) **Advisory**. From time to time important advisory memoranda on various social services are issued by the Department of Health and Social Security. These deal with every aspect of the services including the planning of various residential establishments. Recent examples include advisory memoranda on home helps, community services for the elderly and mentally handicapped and child abuse.

(b) **Policy and planning**. Policy and planning of the social services is an important function of the Department of Health and Social Security. This aspect is particularly essential as many of the plans for the health services depend on simultaneous development of community services. An excellent example is in the case of the services for mentally ill persons who are cared for in mental hospitals. It is hoped to discharge from mental hospital many such people during the next ten years, *but this will be possible only if a parallel increase is provided in all forms of community social services*, including a marked increase in the day centre and hostel provision by local authority social services departments.

Recently the central structure of the Department of Health and Social Security has been reorganized to improve the integration of planning between the social and health services. A central planning division has been set up alongside a central regional division so that in both the social and health services professional officers are closely working with their linked administrative officers. An interesting innovation in the planning of the social services by the Department of Health and Social Security is the 'Regional Plan' introduced for residential services for children under the Children and Young Persons Act 1969. In this, the country is divided into a number of regions and all local authorities within each region co-operate to form a *Regional Planning Committee* under the guidance of the Department of Health and Social Security to ensure that the accommodation planned within the region matches the likely need of the area, as closely as possible.

(c) Financial. This is another important indirect method of control of the social services. Special extra financial allocation is made by the government (acting on the advice of the Secretary of State for Social Services) in the rate support grant (paid by the government to local authorities) so that certain social services can be developed.

Revenue (or costs of running day-to-day services) is financed by

(a) the rate support grant from the government
(b) the local rates.

The *rate support grant* is the large block grant of money paid from the government to local authorities to assist them with their services (it represents approximately 60 per cent of all local government expenditure). It includes a 'population' element and a 'needs' element which reflect the social problems and social services provided by that authority. The actual division of the block grant is made by each local authority (who therefore decides how much will be spent on social services, education, roads, environmental health etc.) However, the larger the rate support grant, the greater the likelihood of social services being developed locally.

Special investigations in the field of social services

The Department of Health and Social Security arranges for special research investigations to be undertaken in the field of social services.

The Secretary of State for Social Security can also, through Parliament, appoint special expert committees to look in detail into certain aspects and to report back.

Rôle of other government departments in social services

Although the main government department dealing with social services is the Department of Health and Social Security, other departments, particularly the *Home Office* and *Manpower Services Commission* do have certain powers.

The **Home Office** is the main department dealing with the problems of law and order in the country and has been active in the encouragement of *community development* in England. This attempts to improve the social conditions of people by encouraging them to participate more in the running of their own affairs. The Home Office has set up a number of interesting seven-year experimental *community development projects* in some cities including Liverpool and Coventry, which could have a very important effect on future social service development.

The **probation service**, run in conjunction with Clerks of the Magistrates, is controlled centrally by the Home Office and a very close link must be maintained between Probation and Social Services Departments especially in relation to the problems and care of delinquent children.

Until 1982, the Home Office also had an important function in social services in the **Urban Aid Programme** (now incorporated into the Inner Areas Partnership, see below). This is a special form of financial aid (both capital and revenue) given to certain projects to encourage new developments, mainly in the large cities and urban areas where there is an urgent need to develop social services. Under Urban Aid the Home Office provides 75 per cent, and the local authority 25 per cent, of the cost. Urban aid covers projects by both local authorities and voluntary bodies, although in the latter instance the appropriate local authority has to pay 25 per cent of the cost of each project. This help usually lasts from 1–5 years. Examples in social services of urban aid projects approved in the last three years include many new day nurseries, day care centres for the elderly, residential units for children and various schemes for the physically and mentally handicapped.

The Manpower Services Commission is mainly concerned with the special employment problems of the handicapped. Its officers include the Disablement Resettlement Officers (see page 213) and the Blind Persons Resettlement Officers. Both work very closely with the social services.

During the past six years, the Department of the Environment has introduced a special '*Inner Area Partnership*' scheme whereby the government has provided 75 per cent of the cost of small capital and revenue projects designed to assist with the rehabilitation of some inner city areas. Most of this money has gone to providing new factories or to improving the physical environment and some to improving social facilities.

The structure of the local authority social services

Following the Local Authority Social Services Act 1970, which was introduced on 1st April 1971, each major local authority must have a Social Services Committee to control its social services (full list given below). Each local authority must appoint a **Director of Social Services** who is the chief officer in charge of the Department of Social Services which administers all the services.

Local authority social services are run by the new County Councils and within the Metropolitan areas (the large conurbations such as Greater Manchester, Merseyside, South Yorkshire, Tyneside, West Midlands, West Yorkshire), by the Metropolitan District Councils, and in London by the London Boroughs. In Scotland, the social work services are controlled by the new Regional local authorities.

Types of social services provided by the Social Services Committees

The following is a summary of services provided by each Social Services Committee:

1 *Care of the elderly*—this includes both field work services carried out within the community, and residential care (see Chapter 16).
2 *Care of the physically handicapped*—blind, deaf and dumb, hard of hearing, spastic, epileptic, paraplegics and other disabled persons (see Chapter 14).
3 *Social work advice to the homeless* (see Chapter 17).
   The main legislation covering these services includes the National Assistance Act 1948 and the Chronically Sick and Disabled Persons Act, 1970.
4 *All child care services* including child care protection, child care supervision, acceptance of parental rights for children committed into the care of the local authority, control of various residential units for children—admission units, reception centres, residential nurseries, children's homes, control of community homes with education on the premises and classifying centres (formerly approved schools and remand homes), and certain services for adoption. Much of the preventive work in non-accidental injury cases is organized under the child care services (see pages 191–96). The legislation for these services is now consolidated into the Child Care Act 1980.
5 *Social work and family casework* dealing with the *mentally disordered* including the provision of social workers (formerly mental welfare officers), adult training centres, workshops and residential accommodation (hostels) for the mentally disordered.
6 *Day care for children under five years of age* including provision of day nurseries and the supervision of private nurseries and child minders.
7 *Provision of home helps.*
8 *Care of unsupported mothers* including residential care.
9 *Hospital social workers*—provision of social work services for hospital patients.

Organization of social services departments

There are many different forms of organization in social services departments. However, most have Area (or District) teams of social workers (see below).

The chief officer is the **Director of Social Services**, next is the Deputy Director of Social Services, and usually an Assistant Director is in charge of the other sections. Each Area (or District) is usually under the control of an Area (or District) social services officer. (A typical arrangement is shown in Figure 12.1.)

It will be noted that there are at least five main parts to the headquarters of a social services department:

1 that dealing with residential services
2 that dealing with field work services
3 that providing facilities for training
4 that dealing with hospital social work.
5 that dealing with administration.

Full details of the various types of residential services are given on the pages mentioned below. In detail these include the following services:

1 **Residential services** for:
   (a) elderly (see page 264)
   (b) children (see pages 187–9)
   (c) physically handicapped (disabled) (see page 211)
   (d) mentally disordered (see pages 241–2)
2 **Field Work services** cover wide types of facilities dealing with:
   (a) family and child care (see pages 183–7)
   (b) disabled (see pages 207–212)
   (c) mentally disordered (see pages 237–243)
   (d) elderly (see pages 250–3)
   (e) transport (see pages 209–210)
   (f) home helps (see pages 266–7)
   (g) meals services—meals-on-wheels or luncheon clubs (see page 251)
   (h) day nursery provision (see pages 181–2)
   (i) homeless families (see pages 268–270)
   (j) adoption services (see pages 197–199)
3 **Training** is provided as follows:
   (a) induction training for new entrants
   (b) in-service training for existing staff
   (c) professional training (field work—social work training), usually by two-year full-time courses
   (d) practical training—receiving students from full-time courses who are doing practical field work placements
   (e) training for residential staff (in both children's units and in old people's homes)
   (f) senior post-graduate training for qualified staff including training in management

The standards of training of social workers is the responsibility of the *Central Council for Education and Training in Social Work* which was established in 1971. This Council is responsible for promotion of training in all fields of social work. At present there are three main ways to train to become a social worker:

1   by obtaining a relevant degree in social sciences and then taking a special one year course;
2   by obtaining any other type of degree and then taking a two year course;
3   by taking a two year course.

Much of this training is carried out in co-operation with universities, polytechnics and commercial colleges run by local education authorities. Each social service department should have a training unit plus training officers.

4   **Hospital social work** deals with the various social problems of patients in hospital. Medical casework is undertaken to help the patient and family to adjust to the illness. Other forms of help and assistance are given with convalescence etc. (see pages 270–271).

Area social services teams

A very important part of each social services department is the *area social services team*. By arranging for all the casework for family and clients to be undertaken by such co-ordinated teams of social workers, it is hoped that problems will be considered as a whole rather than in a fragmented way and that this will lead to a *family social service* dealing with all types of social problem in the family whether this presents as a problem in a child, a disabled person, an old person or a mentally disordered individual.

These teams of social workers are made up of social workers who formerly specialized in child care (with the former children's departments), in mental illness or handicap (previously with the health departments) or with old people or the handicapped (formerly welfare officers of the welfare departments).

The size of areas varies from about 40 000 to 100 000 depending on the district and its social problems. An ideal area will have from ten to thirty social workers mainly working in groups of five or six under the leadership of a senior social worker. Each team deals with the problems of **clients** (the term used for persons referred to the social services department).

Close co-ordination must be maintained with other workers—health visitors, home nurses, medical social workers, teachers, psychiatric social workers, educational welfare officers, community workers, youth leaders, general practitioners and the many voluntary bodies helping in the

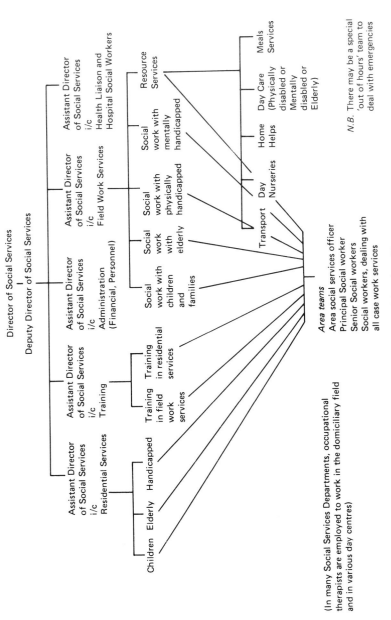

Fig. 12.1 Typical Social Services Department

district. Usually each Area social work team controls the allocation of:

(a) home helps
(b) meals-on-wheels
(c) day nursery places
(d) vacancies in old persons' homes
(e) places in residential accommodation for children
(f) allocation of telephones.

The key individual in each team is the **Area Social Services Officer** and any nurse working in the area who comes across a difficult social problem should refer the case to this officer.

Liaison between the health and social services

It is most important that the closest links are maintained between all medical and social services. Many of the social services in local authorities represent the main supporting services within the community for persons recovering from illness or suffering from some chronic disabling condition. Many of the necessary aids, gadgets or adaptations for the handicapped which are so essential for the successful rehabilitation of many disabling conditions (e.g., arthritis, paraplegia, multiple sclerosis, spasticity, etc.), are supplied by social services departments. The closest possible liaison between the two services must therefore be developed. A map of the Social Services Authorities in England is given in Figure 12.2.

It is very important that liaison between the two services is good. On the health side a community physician is usually appointed with responsibility for liaison—sometimes called a Specialist in Community Medicine (Social Services)—and on the social services side a senior officer is appointed (usually an Assistant Director of Social Services) to take charge of the hospital social work service and to be responsible for integration.

Local arrangements should be made to assist day to day co-operation. Social workers should visit health centres and group practices from time to time so that they can meet not only the general practitioners, but the health visitors, home nurses and school nurses working from the centre.

There should also be working links created between social workers and the hospital services especially through the medical social workers at all hospitals and particularly at geriatric and mental hospitals.

The locally designated community physician responsible for co-ordination acts as medical adviser to the social services department and consequently becomes acquainted with all the medical problems of the department. It is particularly important that *health visitors work closely with social workers* for many of the problems they deal with are also important to the social services department and vice versa. Both health

Fig. 12.2 Social Services Authorities, England

visitors and social workers find themselves working with 'problem families' dealing with different aspects—the health visitor from the preventive health point of view and the social worker dealing with the social difficulties (this is particularly important in preventing non-accidental injury in children—see pages 191–6). The closer that the two groups of officers can work together, the better the results. **Case conferences** are arranged between such workers from time to time to consider difficult individual cases and other officers working with such families are also invited especially those from the education or housing departments. Although the social services department is responsible for the organization of social services within each local authority, co-operation with many different services is needed including those providing health care, education, housing, probation, police and voluntary services. It is only by improving the arrangements between so many different services that the best possible result will be obtained for each family.

13
Care of Children in Need

Local authorities through their social services departments provide help and care to children for a variety of reasons, and, under the Children Act 1975, will have eventually to provide an adoption service.

All Social Service Committees have very special responsibilities through their *child care services* in supervising and looking after children and young persons under the age of 18 years. In much of this work, the social services department is attempting to find *the best possible alternative arrangement for care of the child in the absence of the parents*—either because they have abandoned the child or the child is an orphan or because the parents have been found incapable of looking after the child properly. As will be seen later every attempt is made by trying to settle the child with suitable foster parents so as to provide him with as normal a home as possible. For this reason, large institutional homes are no longer used.

Special help is given to the parent who, because of social reasons, cannot look after his/her child during the daytime. Most of this help is given in *day nurseries or day care centres, playgroups* or *with a child minder*.

Day nurseries

Day nurseries are provided by the Social Service Departments to help care for young children when this cannot be provided at home due to *social circumstances*. Such reasons would include sudden illness of the mother leading to her admission to hospital, or an unmarried mother who has to go out to work to support her family, or a widower or widow with a small child.

Day nurseries open five days a week from early in the morning, 7.30 a.m., to 5.30 p.m. The young child can be brought to the nursery by the parent on the way to work. The child may have all his meals in the nursery and will be completely looked after during the day.

A small charge is made for this service but in priority cases the charge is usually in the region of 40–70 pence per day which is far less than the economic cost. There is no doubt that a day nursery is most useful in helping to care for the children in a family which has to face social difficulties. It avoids having to arrange for the young children to be admitted to a residential home. Day nurseries look after children from a few weeks old up to the age of five years when they can go to school. In some cases, the need for care is temporary while an acute social crisis occurs in the family.

It is usual for about 50 children to be looked after in each nursery. 'Family groups' are set up in each nursery so that about 10 children are looked after together covering an age range from 6 months to 5 years. Babies under 6 months of age are looked after separately.

Each nursery has a trained matron and deputy matron plus a number of trained nursery nurses. The staff are responsible for all aspects of care of the children including their health which must be carefully supervised. Special attention is paid to ensure that:

1   every child is fit when admitted
2   every child is fully immunized
3   any case of communicable disease is immediately investigated.

Dysentery or gastro-enteritis can be particularly serious if they spread in a day nursery (see pages 112–113) and any child with diarrhoea must be sent home until all bacteriological tests are normal.

Day nurseries are being increasingly used for very young handicapped children (with various disabling conditions e.g. spina bifida) to help with their development. It is best if such children are looked after in ordinary day nurseries rather than being segregated in a special nursery. Where a day nursery has a number of handicapped children it will be necessary to employ larger numbers of staff. *Nursery Nurses* qualify after a two year course and by gaining the certificate of the Nursery Nurses Examination Board.

The main clients helped by day nurseries include:

1   the unmarried mother
2   widows or widowers with a young family
3   mothers with a sudden illness
4   parents with a handicapped child especially if the disability is of a type which has led to the child being isolated from the company of other children.

Private day nurseries, playgroups and child minders

Many private day nurseries, playgroups and child minders look after children and each Local Authority through its Social Services Committee is responsible for ensuring that proper standards of staff, fire precautions and accommodation are provided. This is done by insisting that each such unit must be registered with the Local Authority and inspected from time to time to check that the correct standards are being maintained.

Under the Nurseries and Child Minders Regulations 1948, all people caring for more than one child in their own home, whether for profit or not, must be registered with the local authority.

Child care services

These services primarily look after children who need care and protection because of the neglect, abandonment or inability of the parents to cope due to some sudden emergency (illness, separation, etc) or exposure to moral danger. Under the Children Act 1975, in all cases the first consideration is the *need to safeguard and promote the welfare of the child.*

Every social services department *must* investigate fully each case which comes to their knowledge and social workers undertake this inquiry.

In particular there are four main groups of children who need to be looked after:

1 those who have to be cared for by the Social Services Department either because their parents are temporarily absent (such as an illness) or because they have no parents or guardians or because their parents have failed to look after them properly or have abandoned them. The reason may be temporary or permanent and Social Service Departments can either
    (a) receive the children into voluntary care—see below.
    (b) through a court, have statutory care order made which transfers the parental rights to the Social Services Department of the local authority.
2 children and young persons who have been brought before a court for criminal proceedings;
3 children placed by a court in the care of the local authority in connection with matrimonial proceedings;
4 children who have been placed in foster homes or who have been placed privately for adoption.

Child care provisions

Any Local Authority may pass a resolution assuming parental rights over a child if there are no parents or guardians or if the Local Authority considers the parent or guardian unfit to care for that child. If the parents object the matter must be referred to a juvenile court. In practice, in all cases where a Local Authority claims that statutory care is needed (Section 3 Child Care Act 1980) the case is dealt with by a juvenile court.

The types of child care provided by Social Service Departments are either:

1 Voluntary care (a) short-term (less than six months)
                 (b) long-term (more than six months)
2 Statutory care

(1) Voluntary care

This is in many ways similar to voluntary admissions to hospital and is *an informal arrangement* under section (Section 2 Child Care Act 1980). It is used for cases where the social worker is convinced that the circumstances bringing the child into the care of the authority are not serious, i.e. there has not been neglect of the child. Parents can later claim the child when the crisis is over.

There are two main methods of voluntary care:

(a) *short-term care* is used for a sudden family crisis such as an illness, confinement or other sudden emergency. The local authority looks after the child for a short period (never exceeding six months and usually only a few weeks) by the most appropriate method (boarding out, placement in a small home or group home, or even in an admission unit or residential nursery).

Children rarely suffer from much deprivation in such cases and it is usual for other members of the family (parent, brother and sisters) to visit the child;

(b) *long -term care* exceeds six months but is otherwise similar to short-term care. Because of the longer period of care, more permanent arrangements are made for the child which will depend upon the case (see pages 186–7). Once any child has been in voluntary care for 6 months, under Section 56 of the Children Act 1975, any parent must give not less than 28 days notice of intention to remove the child from care. Such notice can be waived by the Local Authority in appropriate cases. Emphasis in long-term care is on *attempting to look after the child in circumstances* which are, as far as possible, *as near those in the child's own home*. For this reason, fostering is ideal or, if this is not possible, placing the child in a family group home containing four to six children of varying ages (resembling a normal family).

(2) Statutory care

This is where a *Court commits the child*, whom it considers is in need of care and protection, *to the care of a local authority*. Such cases are the more serious ones involving grave neglect, abandonment or moral danger to the child. In all such cases the *parental rights are transferred to the local authority*. Once this has happened the only way that the natural parents can reclaim their child is by petitioning the same Court which made the original Order to revoke it. The Court must then decide whether the parents are now responsible enough to justify returning the child to their care. If the Court decides they are not, the child remains in the care of the authority; if the Court decides they are responsible enough, the parents will have the child returned to them.

All neglect, abandonment or moral danger cases are dealt with under the Child Care Act 1980.

Following the Children and Young Persons Act, 1969, a delinquent child found guilty of an offence can be committed to the statutory care of a local authority.

Note: In all cases where parental rights have been transferred to the local authority, these *cease when the young person reaches the age of 18 years*.

Transfer of a child from voluntary to statutory care

Occasionally a child is placed in voluntary care, but his home circumstances deteriorate and the social worker now considers that such an informal arrangement no longer provides sufficient safeguard for the child. In these situations it is possible for the *local authority to assume parental rights* under Section 3 of the Child Care Act 1980. In all such cases, careful rules must be followed by the *local authority* who must always notify the natural parents. This decision by the local authority to assume parental rights can be challenged by the natural parents in the courts.

Children who are victims of divorce

Under the Matrimonial Cause Acts, the High Court can make the local authority *the guardian of the child in a divorce acting under the directions of the court.*

In practice the social services department will then look after the child in the same way as any other child in care (see below).

Child protection

A further safeguard is maintained by social services departments where there is a private agreement or contract between one private individual and another for the placement of a child. In all instances, the social services department of the local authority *must* be notified and it has a *duty* to check that this placement is satisfactory. It must also ensure by subsequent investigation that the child is well looked after.

Cessation of parental rights

In all cases where parental rights have been transferred to the Local Authority, these *cease when the young person reaches the age of 18 years.*

Under the Children and Young Persons Act 1933, a child is defined as a person under 14 years and a young person as one between 14 and 18 years.

Supervision of fostering

When any child is placed with foster parents, it is the duty of the Social Services Department to arrange *regular visiting which must be at not more than six week intervals* (Foster Children Act 1980).

Preventive social and rehabilitation work with children

Increasing emphasis is being laid on the importance of *preventive work in child care.* This depends upon the social services taking action early enough to enable them to prevent a child coming into care or appearing before a Court.

There is a great deal of evidence that everything must be done *to avoid family breakdown.* As this will be made more likely if the family gets into debt and is made homeless, there is power under the Children and Young Persons Act, 1963 for the Social Services Committee to make financial payments to prevent a child coming into care. These may even include the payment of rent arrears. Much of this financial help is concentrated on ways which are likely to prevent child delinquency—holiday adventure schemes or clubs, etc.

The social services department and its social workers should also do all in their power to try *to rehabilitate each child in its care* so that he may eventually return to his family.

Types and methods of child care

The needs of every child should be carefully assessed on admission into care and each child should be placed according to that assessment.

The aim in child care is to look after every child in the way which is best suited to his needs. Supervision is always carried out by trained social workers and each *case must be reviewed every six months* (a duty imposed on all Social Service Departments by the Children and Young Persons Act 1969). The ideal is to care for each child in conditions and environment as near normal as possible.

It is usual for a child first to go to an **Admission Unit** where his special needs are carefully assessed. There are five main ways in which a child can be looked after:

1 *Boarding out of the child with foster parents.* In this case the child lives with the family just as if the child was in his own home. This is an ideal arrangement and is always used wherever possible, particularly with long stay cases. A foster parent may look after one or a number of children and is always very carefully chosen to ensure the right type of person is always used as a foster parent.
    All children in foster care must be visited regularly and at least once

every six weeks by social workers of the social services department and the frequency of such visiting is very carefully controlled by the Department of Health and Social Security. Under the Children Act 1975, a new clause (to be introduced at a future date yet to be determined) will allow any foster parent who has looked after a child continuously for three or more years to insist that the child is only removed with the leave of the court.

2 *Placement of the child in a family group home* containing four to six children of different ages. Wherever boarding out is not possible, this type of care is the next best. It aims to look after the child in small units where life can be very similar to that in any large family. These homes are scattered throughout the community and made inconspicuous so that the child's living conditions can be kept as near normal as possible.

3 *Placement in a small children's home containing from twelve to eighteen children.* Some children do not seem suitable for either boarding out or life in a family group home and these are looked after in small children's homes. Many of the children living in these homes later progress to other forms of care. A certain amount of assessment can be undertaken in such homes and an unstable child often settles well.

4 Very occasionally a child can be placed *in its own home under supervision.* This arrangement is often used during the rehabilitation of a child and to see if he can settle back into a home from which he has had to be removed for some reason in the past.

5 The child may be placed in a children's home run by a voluntary body (such as Barnardos, the National Childrens' Home, etc.).

Need for continuous review

In all instances it is most important *to review each child's progress regularly* and to attempt *to rehabilitate that child* so that eventually it may be possible to return that child to his own home.

With the disturbed child who has had a difficult home background, this may mean many different stages have to be passed through. Such a child may go to a *reception centre, small children's home, boarding out, a short trial back at home* (which may or may not succeed) and much patience is always needed. The eventual success or failure will only be seen when that child becomes an adult; the constant aim is to help children to develop and mature so that they grow into responsible, mature and happy adults.

Community homes

All types of children's homes and the former remand homes and approved schools are now called *community homes.* Some of these have education provided on the premises (see below).

Special residential units

The larger local authorities social services departments usually provide five special residential units—an admission unit, a residential nursery, a reception centre, a community home with education on the premises—for children on remand or for assessment (former remand homes)—and a community home with education on the premises—for treatment (former approved schools).

Admission unit

The admission unit is the place into which all urgent cases are admitted. The number of children looked after varies, but many care for 45–50 children. Children needing short-term care, especially if the emergency is likely to be short lived, are often looked after in admission units but others are carefully assessed in the admission unit to decide which type of care is best suited to the child. Once this has been decided the child goes on to the appropriate care which may be either *residential nursery, reception centre, boarding out* or *admission to a family group or small children's home.*

Residential nursery

Small children under the age of 5 years and babies may be looked after in a *residential nursery* immediately following admission. Many of the short-term care cases will stay there while in care, but some of the older children may later leave for boarding out or other forms of child care.

During the past few years, more and more social service departments have been closing their residential nurseries and relying on using a carefully selected panel of foster parents to look after babies in care. It has been found that such an arrangement is best for it enables a one-to-one relationship to be established between the foster parent and infant.

Reception centre

Some children need a longer period of assessment or may have difficulty in settling down and these are looked after at a *reception centre*. Some of these children are maladjusted and the regime of the centre allows a longer and more expert assessment of the child to be undertaken.

Community homes with education on the premises (for children on remand or for assessment) (CHEs)

Separate community homes are run by the larger Social Services Departments for children on remand or for assessment. Originally their main function was to accommodate children on remand for some serious offence while full investigations (especially psychiatric) took place. Since the Children and Young Persons Act, 1969, *the assessment of each child* who is committed to the care of the local authority by a Court (because of conviction on some serious offence) is an important extra function.

Many children who pass through such community homes are maladjusted or disturbed having come from an unsatisfactory home. It is, therefore, important to have staff in charge who are trained in dealing with such children and each community home should make arrangements for a psychiatrist to be available to help.

Community homes with education on the premises (CHEs)

Entry into such a community home used to follow the decision of a juvenile court sentencing the child. Now the decision in such a case is made by a case conference of social workers of a Social Services Department after assessment at a suitable assessment centre which indicates that a stay in such a community home could be beneficial for the child.

Education for children in care

In all community homes with education on the premises, including admission units and reception centres, the Local Education Authority may run one or two classes at each centre which the children can attend or the teachers may be employed by the Social Services Department.

Once the child is transferred to other types of care—boarding out, family group or small children's homes—the children attend normal schools in the community and, if this is still practicable, the same school that they attended before comming into care.

Juvenile proceedings

A care order under Section 3 of the Child Care Act 1980 (which has the effect of transferring the parental rights from the natural parents to the local authority) may be granted by a juvenile court on the following grounds:

1 that the child is being ill-treated and neglected;
2 that he is exposed to moral dangers;
3 that he is beyond the control of his parent or guardian;

4   that he is of compulsory school age and is not receiving efficient fulltime education;
5   that he is guilty of any offence *excluding homicide* (homicide is dealt with separately by the High Courts).

A juvenile court can only commit a child to the care of the local authority if it is of the opinion that the child needs some extra parental training. The Social Services Department then assesses the child (a process that takes usually 6–8 weeks and may involve psychiatric and psychological examinations). After assessment the Social Services Department may decide to:

1   send the child to a community home with education on the premises;
2   send the child home under supervision;
3   place the child with a foster parent;
4   involve the child in some special type of training such as adventure training etc. (many of these special types of training are available under schemes of *intermediate treatment* provided by arrangement with Children's Regional Planning Committees).

Intermediate Treatment

Following the Children and Young Persons Act 1969, a juvenile court can place a child on a supervision order and attach to it an order for the child to attend a local scheme of *intermediate treatment*. The principle underlying intermediate treatment is that wherever possible it is better to keep the young offender within the family and community and to attempt to resolve problems away from the situation in which they arose. At the same time intermediate treatment aims at:

(a) providing a more realistic method of working with the young offender than removing him or her from home;
(b) avoiding the side effects of institutionalisation which so often may follow placing the young person in a residential home;
(c) avoiding some of the difficulties of reintegration into the community when the child has been admitted to a residential home.

Increasingly intermediate treatment is chosen as an alternative to admitting a child to a Community Home with Education on the premises (CHE). It is usual to arrange that the young person on intermediate treatment undertakes useful tasks such as car maintenance in the hope that his energies will be channelled into the development of skills. A short period of residential care (not longer than a few weeks) may be arranged and wherever possible this is linked to the other programme of help to the young person.

Probation orders

Probation orders for young persons under 17 years have been replaced by *supervision orders* which may be made in both criminal and care proceedings. These supervision orders are now administered by Social Services Departments.

Borstals

The Borstal system of training was introduced in 1908. The aim is to provide training for offenders from 15–21 years of age and the sentence is in two parts: (1) a period of training in a Borstal establishment (run by the Home Office), minimum 6 months, maximum 2 years; (2) a period of supervision up to a further 2 years. Social Service Departments are not responsible for the Borstal system which comes under the Home Office and the Probation service.

Child abuse (including non-accidental injury)

During the past 12 years increasing attention has been paid to the problem of child abuse. This was formerly called non-accidental injury but the term 'child abuse' now used covers deliberate injury to, serious neglect and sexual abuse of a child.

Child abuse is the deliberate injury of children, usually by parents, and is frequently associated with many different factors. In some cases, criminal neglect by parents may be connected with other forms of anti-social behaviour—assaults or drunkenness, but in many instances, frustration, bad living conditions, unsympathetic neighbours or landladies complaining of babies who cry continuously, or psychiatric illness in a parent are the main factors. Parents who themselves were abused as children, are often involved in child abuse. The problem can present itself in many forms but usually starts by one or both parents slapping, hitting, punching or severely shaking the child causing bruises and occasionally more serious injuries. Ill-treatment usually starts gradually but if it is unnoticed, it is quite possible for the child to be seriously injured and it is now estimated that approximately 80–100 deaths per year in children may be caused in this way.

Diagnosis and early recognition

The following may be the first signs of child abuse:

1　Minor bruises which show that the child has been gripped tightly or shaken.

2 Minor injuries (especially facial bruises) probably caused by slapping or hitting the child. The type of injury is usually similar, 70 per cent being soft tissue injuries to the head and face. There may be 'finger bruising' in which the outlines of the fingers which slapped the child are clearly seen within the bruised area. Such bruising tends to pick out the bony prominences. In many cases, the lips are thick and bruised and there is a torn upper lip frenum. Ribs are frequently bruised or broken and X-rays often indicate that these injuries have been caused in the past. Occasionally small burns may be present.

3 An unexplained failure of the child to thrive.

4 Unusual behaviour by the parents. This may take many different forms—over-anxiety and frequent attendance with the child at clinics or surgeries, plausible explanations of an injury which does not fit the case, or unnatural lack of concern for the child's condition.

Child abuse and non-accidental injury are repetitive and progressive

Many cases show similar characteristics; stress of various kinds is common including poverty (in one survey 80 per cent were in receipt of social security), unemployment (many fathers batter their children when engaged in maternal tasks), overcrowding and unsatisfactory housing conditions and many have unstable marriages. Another interesting finding is that the parents are often very young (about four years below the national average). Studies have shown that teenage parents are less tolerant and have a low tolerance towards the baby's crying. A high proportion of the women involved are pregnant at the time.

A proportion of parents shown to be responsible for child abuse are mentally disturbed or inadequate emotionally. It is interesting that the 'innocent' parent (usually the mother) does not do more to protect her child. The most likely explanation is that she has never learnt how to stick up for herself and for their children. Certainly many of the parents involved never received any affection when they were children and consequently find it very difficult to relate as a normal parent does towards their child.

Any additional stress will tend to precipitate problems—moving house often results in much loneliness and resentment and battering is then more likely.

Early diagnosis of child abuse depends upon the alertness of many professional staff including general practitioners, paediatricians, health visitors, district nurses, midwives, social workers and the staff of many voluntary organizations including the NSPCC. Because injury to the child is always a dominant feature, all those working in casualty or accident departments of hospitals should be especially vigilant.

Management and treatment

Once there is a reasonable degree of suspicion of child abuse, the child should at once be admitted to a hospital (or very occasionally a children's home) for diagnosis and for his own safety. In many instances, a *place of safety order* will be obtained from a court or magistrate (this can most easily be arranged by the Social Services Department) but the child may be admitted voluntarily.

In all cases an immediate *case conference* should be arranged which should include those concerned with the immediate case, the paediatrician, general practitioner, health visitor and social worker, as well as the NSPCC and a senior police officer. As the Social Services Department has the statutory duty to protect and care for all children, it is best if the case conference is arranged by the Social Services Department (within 24 hours).

In those instances in which the professional worker does not feel that the suspicions are firm enough to arrange immediate admission to a hospital, it is still advisable to hold a case conference to decide on the next action. If suspicion is very slight, in every instance at least the doctor, health visitor or social worker should:

1   consult the family doctor
2   discuss the details of the case with a senior colleague
3   make a record of such consultations and discussions.

Area Review Committee (Child Abuse)

There is a combined Area Review Committee in each health authority and local Social Services department to act as a policy forming body to ensure that the arrangements in that area for dealing with the problem of child abuse are satisfactory. Each Area Review Committee should include representatives of the appropriate Local Authority (especially the Director of Social Services, who usually acts as the Convenor and Secretary, and the Director of Education), the Health Services (especially paediatric and other consultants, the District Medical Officer, the District Nursing Officer, plus the Specialists in Community Medicine dealing with social services and child health) and a senior police officer, senior inspector of the NSPCC and a representative of the Chief Probation Officer.

Area Review Committees (Child Abuse) should meet regularly (four times per year) and should:

1   Review local practice and procedure for dealing with such cases.
2   Ensure that immediate hospital admission for children at risk is accepted.
3   Approve written instructions defining the exact duties and re-

sponsibilities of professional staff in connection with non-accidental injury.
4   Provide education and training programmes for staff in the health and social services.
5   Review the work of case conferences.
6   Inquire into the circumstances of cases which appear to have gone wrong and from which lessons could be learned.
7   Ensure that procedures are in operation to safeguard continuity of care between neighbouring areas and in those instances when families move to another area.
8   Agree arrangements for the operation of a total register of cases which have been dealt with by case conferences or other action.

Registers

A register of information is essential in each area to ensure there is good communication between the many services involved. Absolute confidentiality is most important and there should also be arrangements to share information between neighbouring authorities. Registers may be set up by voluntary bodies working in this field (e.g. the NSPCC) or by Social Services Departments or by District Health Authorities. The most important feature of registers is that they should be accessible (at all times—on a 24 hour basis) to doctors, nurses and social workers, and that they should include accurate up-to-date information. The ability of a doctor in a casualty department or a health visitor or social worker in the community to seek information from such a register could be vital to early and effective diagnosis of child abuse. Many past serious cases would probably have been prevented had an efficient register been operating in that area enabling early suspicions to be confirmed because a similar incident had occurred before.

Treatment and rehabilitation of known cases of child abuse

Most cases will initially be in the care of the paediatrician who will be responsible for the assessment and treatment of the case in hospital. Assessment should include both physical and psychiatric investigations. Skeletal surveys should be undertaken in doubtful cases. A case conference will be held and should indicate the most likely methods of treatment. These should vary considerably in different cases and will include:

1   Receiving the child into *statutory care* by the local authority (by Court Order). In the very worst cases there will also be prosecution of the parents.

2 Accepting the child into *voluntary care*. (This may be risky in some cases because parents may suddenly remove the child from hospital or children's home. Therefore, in all cases received into voluntary care, the Social Services Department must always be prepared to seek an urgent *Place of Safety Order* if that need arises.)
3 Arranging for the child to remain under supervision in the home by a Court Order.
4 Returning the child home with planned help to the parents.

In all instances the aim is to ensure that the short and long-term interests of the child are met as far as possible. It is important to realize that, although there are a number of serious cases of intentional injury and neglect that can only be properly treated by permanent removal of the child from the parents, the majority of cases are quite different. In these the child abuse has been caused by many other factors—bad living conditions, unemployment, poverty, threat of eviction especially if babies cry repeatedly and by minor psychiatric illnesses. These parents urgently require help and if this can be satisfactorily given they may be assisted to develop into perfectly satisfactory parents and families. However, the causative factors *must* be discovered. In many instances, the temporary provision of residential care (in a residential nursery or children's home) may be required to enable the parent to be treated.

Day care

Many others who have been found to ill-treat their children are very young and often very isolated and lonely. It is usual to find that the mother herself had an unhappy childhood or was brought up in a broken home.

A very useful method of helping is to admit the child to a day nursery or play group and then to arrange for the mother to help in the group. In this way, the mother is assisted to make new friends and to obtain the support she needs. Indirectly she will be taught to improve her relationship with her own child from the example of care she will see in the nursery or play group.

More and more Social Services Departments are now developing day care which can be extended to older children in the same family who come along to the unit after school.

Many girls' schools now arrange for senior girls to help periodically in play groups and day nurseries, and thus to learn more about the methods of care of young children. This is particularly important because more girls now marry before 20 and the incidence of child abuse is highest in teenage mothers.

Some local authorities have arranged to deal with many cases in nurseries close to a paediatric department which makes the development of special working arrangements between the health and social services departments easier.

Periodic review of long-term cases

Some of the most difficult problems are found in long term cases. It is absolutely essential that *periodic reviews* of such cases are undertaken. These must involve the many professional workers who would normally be concerned with the care of that child and especially general practitioners, teachers, school nurses, health visitors, education welfare officers, social workers (including those working in child guidance) as well as those working with voluntary agencies in that area. In all older children (and some of the worst cases of child abuse occur in older children) it is most important that the *levels of communication between teaching staff* and others concerned with the child in school and health visitors and social workers are always good.

The statutory duty to protect and care for all children who are in need is that of the Director of Social Services and his staff. But unless there is an effective network of information between all staff working in education, health and social services, action by the Social Services Department may be delayed until it is too late to prevent further injury. For this reason, long-term cases should never be written off until a case conference agrees that no further risk remains. Unless this multidisciplinary team approach is always used, mistakes of the past will be repeated.

In any serious case of doubt, a doctor or nurse should always arrange immediate hospital admission for the child to enable more detailed investigations to be undertaken. In cases of difficulty, the problem should always be reported by telephone to the Director of Social Services or Area Social Services Officer (see page 178).

Changes introduced by the Children Act 1975

The main purpose of this Act was to reform the existing law in relation to adoption, guardianship and fostering of children. Much of it gives effect to the main recommendations of the Houghton Report.

In addition, an important new principle was introduced by the Children Act, 1975 relating to children both for adoption and in care. In future *there is a duty* for Courts and Local Authorities when making *any decision* about such children:

(a) to have regard to all circumstances but that the first *consideration is the need to safeguard and promote the welfare of the child*;
(b) to find out as far as possible *the wishes and feelings of the child* and to give due consideration to them.

This means that the needs of the child must take pride of place over all other considerations, i.e. the child's needs are more important than the needs of the natural parents.

Adoption services

Every Social Service Authority (County Councils, Metropolitan Districts and London Boroughs) eventually must establish and maintain *an adoption service*. This should be done in conjunction with its other social services for children and with the other approved societies in its area. In future therefore all Social Services Committees will be in charge of an adoption service.

The responsibility for approval and registration of adoption societies in England and Wales was transferred to the Secretary of State for Social Services. It is hoped that this will ensure uniformly good standards of adoption practice throughout the country.

The legal status of an adopted child will, in future, be exactly similar to a child born to the adopters.

Unless the child is related to the adopters or has been placed with them by a High Court order or an adoption agency, an adoption order cannot be made unless the child has had his home with the applicants for at least 12 months.

The following are some of the more important requirements for adoption:

1 Legal adoption is by an *adoption order* granted by a Court of Law.
2 Persons who may adopt must be at least 21 years of age.
3 Adoption must be in the best interests of the child.
4 Adopters must live within the UK, the Channel Islands or the Isle of Man.
5 A married person cannot apply on her own unless her husband
   (a) cannot be found;
   (b) is permanentaly separated from her; or
   (c) is incapable of joining in the application because of mental or physical illness.
6 A parent and step-parent will not normally be able to get an adoption order if the parent has been given custody of the child following divorce. The applicants are directed back to the divorce court so that that court may consider the situation including that of the step-parent in the custody arrangements.
7 A sole father or mother—the court cannot make an order in favour of a mother or father alone unless:
   (a) the other natural parent is dead or cannot be found; or
   (b) there is another reason justifying the exclusion of the other natural parent.

8   Normally a male person cannot adopt a female child.
9   Adoption must NOT be arranged for reward.
10 During the adoption process, the court appoints a *Guardian ad litem*
    who is an officer appointed to safeguard the interests of the child on
    behalf of the Court. It is usual for certain social workers in the Social
    Services Department to act as *Guardian ad litem* officers.

Parental consent to adoption

Important new changes were made in arrangements for parental consent
by the Children Act 1975. At a date to be decided in the future, parental
consent to adoption (by the natural parent) will be given *before* the
adoption order is made. A natural parent *will agree to free the child for
adoption.* This will remove the present unsatisfactory uncertainty for all
adopters and also will stop the natural mother from having to re-affirm
her consent a number of times (this can be very harassing for any natural
mother).

Ground for dispensing with parental consent

Parental consent can now be dispensed with if the parent or guardian has
seriously ill-treated the child and, because of the ill-treatment, the
rehabilitation of the child within the household of the parent or guardian
is unlikely.

Religion

In future adoption agencies *as far as is practicable* must respect the
parents' wishes in regard to the religious upbringing of the child. (This
replaces the present system of parental consent to adoption subject to the
condition that the child is brought up in a particular faith.)

Courts

At present adoption proceedings are held usually in Juvenile Courts. The
Children Act 1975 enables *at some future date* adoption proceedings to be
transferred from Juvenile Courts to domestic magistrates courts.
    It is most important in all adoptions that:

    (a) as far as possible, a careful matching process is carried out so that
every effort is made to place the child with applicants who have similar
intellectual, economic, cultural and religious background as the natural

parents. Careful matching does much to ensure that the child is adopted by parents from a similar background and with similar educational attainments as the natural parents of the child.

(b) a careful medical history is taken of all children who are likely to be adopted and also of all prospective adopting parents.

The general health of the child should be good and every effort should be made to ensure the child has no serious defects of sight, hearing, speech or congenital abnormality. Mental handicap should be carefully tested for (as far as is practicable). Serological tests for syphilis should always be carried out.

The health of the prospective adopting parents should likewise always be carefully considered. They both should be in good general health, be suitable temperamentally and psychologically to care for a child. There should also be a good family history. In particular, the medical conditions which would cause doubt about the suitability of anyone to be a prospective adoptor would include a history of mental illness, mental handicap, epilepsy, tuberculosis and any serious chronic illness.

Access to birth records

Adopted persons over *the age of 18 years have now a legal right to* information about their birth records. Section 26 of the Children Act 1975 lays this down and places upon local authority Social Services Departments and adoption agencies *a duty to provide counselling.* Those adopted after 12 November 1975 will be given an opportunity to see a counsellor *but need not do so.* Those adopted before 12 November 1975 must *see a counsellor* before they are given the information they seek.

Custodianship

A new legal status called 'custodianship' was introduced by the Children Act 1975 and it will come into operation at a future date yet to be decided. This is meant to be an alternative to adoption and could be described as a half-way stage between adoption and fostering. Legal custody is transferred but the child keeps his name, and his family contacts are not cut off.

Custodianship can be granted by the Court on an application of a relative, step-parent or any other person who is not the father or mother of the child but who has the child in his care. Usually parental consent is necessary, and in addition

1   the child must have had his home with the applicant for at least three months in the case of relatives and step-parents;

2   and for all other applicants the child must have had his home there for
    at least 12 months.

Custodianship can be *granted without parental consent* in two
circumstances:

(a) where there is no person having legal custody of the child, or
(b) when the child has had his home with the applicant for at least three
years.

All applicants for custodianship must give notice to the local Social
Services Department who then must investigate and report to the Court.
However where applicants have looked after the child for at least three
years or more (as in the case of long-term foster-parents) *that child* cannot
be removed from their care without leave of the Court (section 41,
Children Act, 1975). This is designed to prevent the 'tug-of-love'
situations from developing where a foster parent who has had the child
for three years or more wishes to keep the child although the Social
Services Department who has parental rights wishes to remove the child
for some reason. In future in such a case the foster-parent will be able to
keep that child *while a Court decides on any custodianship application.*

14
Care and Rehabilitation of Disabled People

The Department of Health and Social Security is centrally responsible for the community social services for disabled or physically handicapped people.

Locally each major local authority (County Council, Metropolitan District Council or London Borough) is responsible through its Social Services Committee and the chief officer in charge of these services is the Director of Social Services (see page 175).

In addition, there are large numbers of national and local voluntary bodies working for the handicapped; examples include the Royal National Institute for the Blind, The Royal Association for Disability and Rehabilitation (RADAR), the National Spastics Society, the national Multiple Sclerosis Society, and various Deaf and Dumb Associations, etc. Most local authorities give monetary grants to help such voluntary bodies.

Relationships between medical and nursing services and social services

Medical, nursing and social services all attempt to help the handicapped in different ways. Doctors and nurses carry out the physical treatment of the handicapped in hospitals or in the community while the social services are more concerned with rehabilitation and with helping them to lead an active life and to overcome their social problems or difficulties. It will follow from this that doctors, nurses and social workers must work closely together if the best results are to be obtained. The fact that the local areas of operation for each are roughly the same geographical size helps to ensure that the closest liaison can usually be achieved.

Generally social services concentrate upon *aids to normal life within the community*—upon *housing, adaptations to houses, employment, special workshops, transport, various aids and gadgets, handicraft centres, social centres* and *clubs* and *holidays*. For these reasons, most social services provided by local authorities are in the community while many medical and nursing services are in the hospital or outpatient departments. Home nurses, health visitors and general practitioners also are actively engaged in helping many handicapped in their own homes. It is *most important that the social worker links up with these medical and nursing services*; this is best done by social workers visiting hospitals and general practitioners to ensure that a continuous working arrangement is maintained at all times. The eventual success with any individual handicapped person is closely connected with the degree of such co-operation between doctors, nurses and social workers. Eventually it is hoped that social workers will work closely with primary health care teams.

Legislation

Disabled Persons (Employment) Acts, 1944 and 1958

These Acts are designed to help all disabled people. Their names are held on a register and all employers are required to maintain a minimum percentage of disabled people among their employees.

A '*disabled person*' is one 'who on account of injury, disease or congenital deformity, is substantially handicapped from obtaining or keeping employment'. Every employer who employs twenty or more people must, under this Act, employ a *minimum of 3 per cent of disabled persons* among his staff.

Although the wide definition of disabled people has reduced the effectiveness of this Act, it has helped to increase the opportunities for employment of handicapped people.

Chronically Sick and Disabled Persons Act, 1970

The Chronically Sick and Disabled Persons Act, 1970 gives many special responsibilities to local authorities in respect of those who are substantially and permanently handicapped (including those who are mentally handicapped). The main duties of local authorities are:

(1) Information. Local authorities must ensure (*a*) that they are adequately informed of the numbers and needs of the handicapped so that they can properly plan and develop their services, and (*b*) that the handicapped and their families know what help is available to them by general publicity and personal explanations.

(2) Provision of services. Local authorities, when satisfied that the following services are necessary to the handicapped person, can provide the following:

   (a) Practical assistance in the home
   (b) Wireless, television, library or similar recreational facilities in the home

(c) Recreational facilities outside the home and assistance in taking advantage of educational facilities

(d) Travelling facilities for handicapped persons

(e) Assistance in carrying out adaptations to the home

(f) Facilitating the taking of holidays

(g) Meals at home or elsewhere

(h) A telephone and any special equipment necessary for its use.

(3) Housing. Every local authority must have regard to the special needs of the disabled and any new houses planned must show that special provision is made for them. This clearly gives housing authorities a duty to plan and provide special housing accommodation for handicapped people.

(4) Premises open to the public. There are a series of requirements for public buildings. These deal specially with:

(a) Providing means of access to and within the buildings and in the parking facilities and sanitary conveniences for the disabled. Such provision must be considered before planning permission is given.

(b) Need for a local authority to provide public sanitary conveniences for disabled people.

(c) Need for anyone providing sanitary conveniences in premises open to the public for accommodation, refreshment or entertainment, to make provision, as far as is practicable, for the disabled.

(d) Adequate sign-posting for the above provisions from outside.

(e) Need to provide facilities for access, parking, sanitary conveniences suitable for the disabled as far as is practicable at school, university and other educational buildings.

In addition, there are special clauses about Advisory Committees for the handicapped either nationally or locally and these insist that members of such committees must include persons with experience of work for the disabled and people who are themselves disabled.

Many local authorities have provided excellent new services (especially telephones) for the handicapped, but some have been slow to assist. As some of the more progressive local authorities provide these extra services free and others make charges, there is unfortunately a varying standard of service for the handicapped throughout the country.

National Assistance Act, 1948, Section 29

This gives the local authorities the responsibility of providing a further wide range of social services for handicapped people including home training, occupational therapy and many other domiciliary services.

General principles for helping disabled people

In the rehabilitation of all these groups of handicapped people, there are certain basic principles which are important. No social service can succeed if they are ignored, and it is essential to understand them, for they carry the secret of success and can quite simply be modified for every handicapped person. There are four main principles:

1   The problems of every handicapped person are *highly individual* and *personal*;
2   The best solution for any handicapped person is that *one which is as near normal as possible*;
3   A large amount of *improvisation* will probably be necessary;
4   *Great determination and singleness of purpose* is usually essential for success.

1   The difficulties of any handicapped person vary with each individual. This is because the problems depend on:

   (a) the age of the person
   (b) the nature and extent of the handicap
   (c) the reaction of the disabled person to the handicap

Thus, many blind people are able to hold down an important job whilst others who are blind may be unable to carry out successfully quite a simple occupation. The handicap is the same—complete blindness—but the end result and size of the individual problem varies greatly. Age also is an important factor (see page 214).

The reaction of handicapped people to these difficulties depends very much on the attitude of those who have tried to help in the early and crucial stages. A correct approach and attitude of mind here are essential. What is wanted is an understanding, which very often means something quite different from ineffective and maybe sentimental sympathy. Usually often the best approach is a fairly tough one which promises the handicapped person little but many hard struggles and disappointments.

For these reasons, *individual visiting* and *assessment* are always a most important first step in rehabilitation. As the social background of the handicapped person—his home and his family—will always play a significant part in overcoming the handicap, it is important that assessment includes these.

2   There is a very simple rule to follow in determining what any handicapped person should attempt to do. *The best solution is always the one which is as near normal as possible.*

This basic principle applies to all aspects of work with handicapped people including education and occupation. A normal person works in an industry or in an office with normal people—he is not in any way protected. This is also the best solution for any handicapped person.

If difficulties are found in suggesting the next stage in rehabilitation, a useful indicator is given by considering what occupation the person would be following if he was not handicapped. The aim should always be for the rehabilitation process to progress towards this goal.

The constant hope given by successfully reaching various stages in rehabilitation will do much to counteract an attitude of self pity in the handicapped person which, at all cost, must be avoided.

3 Just as the problems of each handicapped person differ, so will the solutions. Hence, an ability *to improvise* in overcoming the inevitable and unexpected difficulties is most important. Those working with handicapped people cannot afford to be narrow minded, too set in their ways or hidebound by convention. All the most successful are resilient and often unconventional people to whom improvisation comes naturally.

4 It is always easy to find an excuse for failure when dealing with handicapped people. Therefore, to succeed, it is important to *concentrate solely upon success* however remote this might seem to be. If possible, the handicapped person and those immediately around him, should be fired with an enthusiasm to succeed irrespective of the difficulties and inevitable disappointments ahead. A complete singleness of purpose should be encouraged and this often helps to overcome difficulties.

Main groups of disabled

The main groups of disablement for which local authorities provide social services include:

1 Blindness and partial sightedness
2 Total deafness from birth—including the deaf and dumb
3 Hardness of hearing—acquired deafness, usually late in life
4 Congenital disabilities—spina bifida or spastic diplegia
5 Paraplegia and hemiplegia
6 Various paralytic diseases—multiple sclerosis, muscular dystrophy, poliomyelitis
7 Strokes
8 Serious arthritic conditions—rheumatoid arthritis, spondylitis, severe osteoarthritis
9 Epilepsy
10 Accident cases

Special financial help available to seriously disabled people

Attendance allowance

Attendance allowance is an allowance for adults and children aged 2 years and over who are severely disabled physically or mentally and have needed a lot of looking after for 6 months or more. There are two rates, the higher rate for those who require attendance both by day and night (£27.50 in 1983) and a lower rate for those who need attendance either by day or night (£18.15 in 1983). The allowance is NOT payable if the disabled person is living in accommodation provided by a local authority or is receiving free in-patient treatment in a National Health Service hospital.

A kidney patient on dialysis is paid the allowance if dialysis takes place at home, but not if it is carried out in hospital for more than 4 weeks.

Mobility allowance

The mobility allowance is a cash benefit which is payable to seriously disabled persons aged 5–65 to help them become more mobile. Anyone of 65 in receipt of a mobility allowance may continue to receive it until 75. New applicants, however cannot qualify after the age of 65. It is additional to any other social security benefit, is taxable but for married women is considered as part of her 'earned income' and therefore usually, in such cases, is exempt from tax. In 1983 it was £18.30 a week.

To qualify, the applicant must live within the UK and have resided there for at least 12 months within the preceding 18 and the following special medical conditions must be satisfied:

1   the person must be unable or virtually unable to walk because of physical disablement, *and*
2   the inability to walk must be likely to persist for at least 12 months from the time the claim is made, *and*
3   the person's condition must be such that he can benefit from time to time from increased facilities for mobility.

The mobility allowance is paid to more than one person who qualifies living in the same household. It is intended to aid mobility but may be used for any purpose—helping to pay for the family car, hiring taxis, taking a holiday etc. In the case of an adult receiving the allowance on behalf of a child, that person then has to sign an undertaking to apply the allowance for the benefit of the disabled child.

Motability

This is the name of a voluntary organization formed on the initiative of the government to assist disabled persons to get maximum value for money in using their Mobility Allowance to acquire a car. Two schemes are available:

1   a leasing scheme;
2   a hire purchase scheme.

In the first, a new car is leased for 3–4 years in return for surrendering the mobility allowance for this period and also paying a 'once and for all' advance rental (from £173 for Mini 1000 HL Manual—1982). Full details of both schemes can be obtained from RADAR, Mortimer Street, London W1.

Exemption from vehicle excise duty (VED)

All recipients of the mobility allowance are exempt from the VED. This also applies to *those who qualify but are over the age limit.*

Social services available for disabled people

The following are the social services provided by local authority social services departments and voluntary bodies working with them:

(1) Social worker support and assessment

Social workers are available to assess and advise the handicapped at home. Initially each handicapped person is **registered** and his/her needs carefully assessed and catalogued. Social workers are usually attached to area social work teams (see page 176) and include specialists trained to work with the blind who can teach Braille and with the deaf and dumb who can use sign and finger language.

Social workers work closely with other community workers such as health visitors, home nurses and general practitioners. Special services such as meals-on-wheels and home helps can be arranged by the social worker.

(2) Employment for disabled people

There are two main ways in which disabled people can be employed full time: (*a*) in ordinary or 'open' industry, (*b*) in special sheltered employment.

(*a*) *'Open' industry* refers to ordinary occupations where each handicapped person works with and under exactly the same conditions as a normal person. Full wages are paid without any subsidy.

This is always the best solution, but is unfortunately only possible for a proportion of the employable handicapped. The success of placing a handicapped person in open industry will depend on the employment opportunities of the area and the efforts of the social services department and Disablement Resettlement Officers (DROs) of the Employment Services Division of the Manpower Services Commission to find openings in local industries. It should be possible to place many intelligent well trained disabled persons in most industries. With the blind, *special Blind Persons Resettlement Officers* are employed to assist finding places in industry for the handicapped (see page 216).

(*b*) *Sheltered employment* is subsidized employment (full-time) arranged either in a special workshop or in a home workers scheme (details for the blind on pages 214–19). The Employment Services Division runs special Remploy workshops for handicapped people and some local authorities run their own workshops. There are also many voluntary bodies who run sheltered workshops usually with financial help from local authorities.

(3) Industrial therapy services

Many local authorities run industrial therapy services and, in this way, assist the handicapped with their rehabilitation. Reference is made later to such services provided for mentally handicapped people (see pages 240–41) and similar services are provided for the physically handicapped. The aim of these services is mainly to train and prepare physically disabled individuals for full-time work.

(4) Handicraft centres

Handicraft centres are also provided by local authorities for disabled people and are usually staffed by handicraft instructors. The main aim of such centres is to assist those who are disabled to enjoy recreational facilities although complete rehabilitation towards eventual full-time employment may not be possible.

(5) Occupational therapy services

Most local authority social services departments employ occupational therapists. These may be on a *domiciliary basis* where the occupational therapist calls on each handicapped person at home from time to time, or the services may be provided at *special rehabilitation centres.* In such cases the handicapped persons are brought to the centre by special transport.

The concept of the work of occupational therapists has changed and *much more emphasis is now placed on teaching disabled people to live with their handicaps* rather than instruction in craft work. In this way they are helped to overcome their muscular difficulties by the use of various aids or machines including knitting and fretsaw machines, various looms and treadle lathes. A number of crafts are also taught at such centres.

Occupational therapists also train patients in *special training kitchens* and these are especially useful to the handicapped housewife to help her become more independent. Various aids and gadgets are tested out in these kitchens so that later the correct aid can be fitted in each handicapped person's own kitchen.

Attendance at such centres may be on a full-time or part-time basis. As well as the training undertaken at each centre, the social value of handicapped people meeting each other and becoming less isolated is also important.

Much chronic invalidism can be caused by the disabled person becoming more and more withdrawn as he/she stays permanently at home meeting only close friends or family. If the handicapped person is brought to a rehabilitation or handicraft centre, his/her confidence is helped by meeting other people and seeing what can be achieved, and further deterioration can be prevented. Domiciliary occupational therapy services are also provided by many health authorities.

(6) Aids centres

Permanent aids centres containing a wide range of equipment suitable for the disabled have been established in London by the Disabled Living Foundation and by some local authorities including Liverpool, Newcastle and Birmingham. These aids centres set out to enable disabled people and their families to see for themselves the range of equipment available. It is usual to staff such units with experienced occupational therapists and to run the centre on an appointment system as it usually takes $1\frac{1}{2}$ to 2 hours to demonstrate all the equipment available.

Disabled people and their families wishing to visit such centres should contact either the Disabled Living Foundation, 346 Kensington High Street, LONDON W8, or the local Directors of Social Services.

(7) Transport

Mobility for handicapped people is very important. Individual problems depend very much on the type of handicap. Various adaptations can be made to cars so that they can be safely driven by hand controls only.

Individual transport. Individual transport for severely disabled people is the responsibility of the government. Until 1976, direct provision of adapted cars or three-wheelers (Invacars) was the main method. But direct provision, through the Artificial Limb and Appliance Service, is now available only to war pensioners and very special cases. All other severely handicapped persons use the mobility allowance (see page 206). The production of Invacars has ended but stocks will allow those who have such a vehicle to obtain a replacement until approximately, 1983. After that date such persons (and all new applicants) must rely on the mobility allowance. Anyone using an Invacar may transfer to the mobility allowance without medical examination or age limit.

Local authorities provide the run-in, drive and base for the garage which is erected by the Department of Health and Social Security.

Local authorities often provide *temporary* wheelchairs on loan to help those who have a transient need—less than six months. In permanent cases, after this period, the Artificial Limb and Appliance Service should provide the wheelchair.

Group transport. Local authority social services departments provide various vehicles, *personnel carriers, mini-buses*, etc., to carry to handicapped from their homes to various centres. Many of the vehicles are fitted with *side hydraulic lifts* so that wheelchairs and their occupants can easily be loaded onto them while sitting in their wheelchair. At their destination, the chair and occupant can likewise be easily unloaded.

The success of many of the activities and services provided by local authorities (various centres and clubs, etc.) depends to a large extent on the efficiency of transport services for handicapped people which must be adequate to meet the needs of the area.

(8) Holidays and outings

Many voluntary bodies and local authorities arrange special holiday schemes for disabled persons. These have become more and more ambitious in recent years and include special holidays abroad.

Special staff go with the handicapped group which usually contains many quite severely handicapped people in wheel chairs. Special arrangements are made as regards transport and all holiday activities, and in this way, many handicapped people are able to enjoy a holiday who otherwise could not do so.

Some local authorities also help handicapped people by subsidizing ordinary holidays arranged by the disabled person himself/herself with a small monetary grant. This enables the disabled person to arrange a more expensive type of holiday (e.g. to stay at a hotel with a lift).

Emphasis today is on the *provision of normal holidays* in which the normal members of the family can share with the disabled individual. There are, however, a number of special holidays arranged for handicapped people and some local authorities have special seaside holiday homes for the disabled.

(9) Social centres and clubs

Many voluntary bodies run special social centres and clubs for handicapped people. Local authorities usually give financial support to such centres or provide a central club which voluntary bodies may use at no cost. Transport can be provided by the local authority.

(10) Housing for disabled people

The *design of the home occupied by the individual disabled person is very important.* Many adaptations are needed to enable a severely handicapped person to live normally—larger doors, no steps, large bathrooms and WCs and special fitments.

It may be possible to *adapt the home* or to introduce special aids (see below). But with the most severely handicapped, e.g., the paraplegic, it may be easier and cheaper for the local housing authority to *build specially designed bungalows* which incorporate such adaptations.

In the case of an individual who suffers a paraplegia following an accident and who is consequently admitted to a regional hospital spinal centre, *it is most important that the housing requirements are considered shortly after admission* and not left until just before the patient is discharged home. Most patients will remain in such hospitals for at least six months and it is essential to ensure that the local authority has all this time to solve the housing difficulties which often are considerable. Certain considerable adaptations may be needed at the patient's home or even rehousing—either of which may take months to achieve.

(11) Minor adaptations, aids and gadgets

Under the Chronically Sick and Disabled Persons Act, 1970, local authorities help by providing (usually at no cost) minor adaptations including:

1 *Ramps or handrails.*
2 *Hoists* in bedrooms and bathrooms for those paralysed in the legs so that they can become more independent and mobile.
3 *Modifications to table implements*, knives, forks, spoons, to make them more easily used by people whose grip is weak or whose hands are deformed.

4 Various *kitchen fitments for handicapped people.* These include many gadgets for one-handed people or those who only have power in one hand, and other aids for those whose balance is poor (slings to be fitted to sinks to allow such people to stand supported by the sling);

5 *Kitchen management and planning* is most important. The height of various working surfaces and the design of kitchen furniture are examples. Many rehabilitation centres are fitted with *model kitchens* for handicapped people so that the occupational therapist can see which equipment best suits the handicapped person before steps are taken to fit out the handicapped person's own kitchen. Various kinds of cooking stoves can be tried in such demonstration kitchens.

6 Various *personal aids in dressing* are all important so that the independence of the handicapped person is improved. In all this work, the aim is always to make the handicapped person as normal as possible and, in this respect, anything that engenders independence is valuable.

Other social services which are available include meals-on-wheels (see page 251) and home helps (see page 266) for which charges are usually made.

Telephones. Under the Chronically Sick and Disabled Persons Act, 1970, most local authorities help by providing a telephone (and paying rent) for those who are severely handicapped and who live alone. Standards vary but most local authorities give top priority to the handicapped living alone who cannot go outside even in fine weather. Telephones are also provided for special medical cases. Any nurse coming across such a handicapped person who urgently requires a telephone should report the case to the local Director of Social Services.

Rehabilitation of disabled people

This is a joint enterprise involving the medical services (hospitals and general practitioners), Employment Services Division and local authority social services departments and, in children and young persons, the education authority.

Rehabilitation usually starts in the hospital—in the rehabilitation or orthopaedic departments and then transfers to rehabilitation centres run by local authorities or special hospitals. Special transport is used to bring the patient to the centre and makes it possible to extend more quickly the range of rehabilitation.

At the centre, there are many and various machines and aids such as knitting machines, fretsaw machines, looms, as well as a training kitchen. There are also opportunities to follow many crafts.

The rehabilitation centre is usually open all day and people can attend for half a day or a full day. It is usual for the kitchen to be used by a handicapped person learning to cook, and in this way meals are prepared for themselves and others attending the centre. One of the most valuable parts of the centre's regime is the *social one*, whereby handicapped people meet others. In many long and chronic illnesses or disabilities, there is a strong tendency for the patient to become more and more withdrawn and tends to stay permanently at home meeting only the family and close friends who call. Even when the physical disability improves, the individual very often tends to stay at home and this factor can have the effect of making it difficult or impossible to rehabilitate the person back to an occupation.

Attendance at the occupational therapy centre and travelling to it increases greatly self-confidence and does much to prevent permanent invalidism. Once a week at the centre, a social evening is arranged so that those attending the centre can relax together playing games, table tennis and dancing.

Rehabilitation from centre to workshops and industry

The aim of the occupational therapist is to transfer eventually the handicapped person either directly into *open industry* or to a *special sheltered workshop*. These are run by social service departments, various voluntary bodies supported by local authorities by financial grants and by the Employment Services Division through the special Remploy factories. These workshops are sited throughout the country and are designed to provide permanent work for the severely disabled person.

Another very important link in the rehabilitation chain is the Employment Rehabilitation Centres run by the Training Services Division. These are designed to teach a handicapped person a new trade skill and are of great importance to those people who have had to learn a new job because the one for which they are trained is now unsuitable for them. An example would be a skilled miner who had a serious accident. Even though he may be left with only a minor degree of disability, it is obviously unwise for him to return to mining. Therefore, he is retrained at such a centre and is given a new industrial skill. This is most essential as it is the industrial skill of the handicapped person that usually determines whether he can be employed or not. The *highest unemployment rate is always in the unskilled workers*. If, therefore, in addition, there is a history of physical handicap, their chance of employment may be very slight. For this reason, *all handicapped people should be taught an industrial skilled occupation* suitable to their handicap, and the Centre is equipped to do this.

There must, at all times, be complete co-ordination between the occupational therapist and the Disablement Resettlement Officer.

Detailed social services for disabled people

Blind and visually handicapped (including partially sighted)

Registration

Proper registration is essential. Anyone who is thought to be blind is examined by a consultant ophthalmologist who carries out a complete visual examination and indicates, in his report, the degree of lack of sight and the prognosis.

Expert examination is most important to make certain that further active treatment is not possible, and to obtain an accurate knowledge of the number of blind persons present, their ages and requirements.

At present there are approximately 105 000 persons registered in England and Wales. Of these 85 per cent are aged 50 years and over. So, the problem of blindness mainly occurs in late middle-aged and elderly persons.

Just over 11 000 new cases of blindness are registered each year. There is a marked increased incidence of blindness in women compared with men. There is an even more marked tendency among the newly blinded to be elderly as only 8 per cent of the newly blinded are under 50 years of age and 81 per cent of them are aged 65 years and over.

Because of the close association between blindness and old age, it must always be remembered that many of the problems discussed in Chapter 16 on the elderly may also present major difficulties for them.

Individual assessment

The problems facing any blind person vary greatly from individual to individual. The age at which blindness develops is a major factor. The child born blind has to learn to live the whole of his life as a blind person—being educated as a blind person, employed as a blind person and face the difficulties of retirement and old age with the same handicap. Many elderly persons going blind over the age of 70 have only the last years of their life to lead as blind people—education and employment never present any difficulties. In the intermediate group there obviously are different problems.

The *personality, past training, intelligence* and the *home conditions* will all have a marked effect on either reducing or increasing the difficulties facing the blind person.

Each blind person must be carefully and individually assessed by expert social workers (usually called *home teachers for the blind*) whose task it is to unravel each problem and arrange for help.

As already explained, the attitude of the social worker can do a great deal to minimize the difficulties of each blind person.

With newly blinded adult people (rather than with aged newly blinded), assessment is never easy, for often the blindness has suddenly occurred leaving the person uncertain, full of self-pity and maybe bitter. Such newly blinded people should always be sent to a *special assessment centre* such as the one at Queen Elizabeth Homes of Recovery, Torquay, which is run by the Royal National Institute for the Blind. Here, under expert guidance, the newly blinded person spends from four to six weeks while being assessed. Any self-pity is quickly lost and the individual soon realizes that life as a blind person can still be full and interesting. After a visit to this home, most newly blinded people return home and approach the necessarily difficult period of industrial retraining with a new and essential spirit of hope.

Even when the blind person has settled down well, *periodic home visits should be paid by a trained social worker* to continue in an unobtrusive way the assessment of current problems. Only in this way is it possible to ensure that the wide social services available to blind people are being properly used.

Employment

About 16 per cent of the blind people in this country are between the ages of 16 and 60 years, and it is in this group that the problem of employment occurs.

Full time employment of blind people includes:

1 Employment in 'open-industry'
2 An occupation in sheltered employment:
   (a) in workshops
   (b) in home workers schemes.

(1) Employment in 'open industry'. The term 'open industry' is used to denote employment in an ordinary job (in industry or commerce) where the blind person works with sighted people. No special arrangements are made as regards remuneration, for the blind person in open industry is exactly like other sighted workers.

There are many different types of occupations in which the intelligent, highly trained blind person can make a success, including a number of industrial processes such as capstan lathe operatives, telephone operators, piano tuners, etc.

The placing of blind people successfully in open industry depends on:

(a) having a helpful and sympathetic employer who is prepared to try out one or two blind people
(b) being able to train the blind person not only before the job starts but actually while carrying it out.

In both respects, the work of the *Blind Persons Resettlement Officers* of the Employment Services Division is invaluable. These officers include very highly trained blind persons who arrange for the placement of blind people in industry. They liaise with the employers and find out what vacancies exist locally, in open industry, which would be suitable for blind people. The Resettlement Officer then assesses the potential of the blind persons wishing to enter open industry and trains those selected. The officer then introduces each blind person to his new post and stays to help and train him. In this way, this officer is able to guide the blind person through the most difficult part of the job—the beginning, and help in the settling down period. Afterwards visits are paid to the factory from time to time to check how the blind person is doing. If any difficulties occur in the meantime, the employer can call upon the Blind Persons Resettlement Officer to help sort them out. There is no doubt that this service helps many blind people to find out and maintain employment in industry.

On the general principle already mentioned, *the aim should always be to try and place as many blind people as possible in 'open industry'*—an employment solution which is normal. It is encouraging to note, in many areas, a steady increase in the proportion of blind people in open industry. In some areas, the proportion of blind people in open industry is in excess of 65 per cent of blind people employed full-time.

(2) Occupation in sheltered employment. For those blind people who cannot for some reason manage to hold down a job in 'open industry', the next alternative is to try and place them in what is known as 'sheltered employment'. This is specially subsidized full-time occupation applicable to blind persons only.

(a) If possible, the blind person needing sheltered employment should be sent to a special workshop for the blind. Here, after a period of training in a suitable occupation, he is employed in the workshop. There are many traditional trades for blind persons in workshops including basket making, rug making, brush making, chair caning, machine knitting.

Each blind person attends the workshop full time just as in an ordinary factory and is employed there. Specially trained sighted foremen assist them in the finishing-off of articles, and arrange the marketing and sale of the products.

Each blind worker receives the usual wage for the occupation although because of his handicap he might not have been able to earn his wage 'on piece rates'. The difference between what is actually earned and is paid is called 'augmentation' and is paid by the local authority.

Provided certain conditions are met, the Employment Services Division will make a grant equal to 75 per cent of the financial deficiency each year to the authority for each approved worker in sheltered employment. Certain capital grants are also available to voluntary bodies who provide satisfactory sheltered employment.

(b) Home workers schemes are mainly to be found in rural areas and smaller towns where it is never possible to collect enough blind people together to form a sheltered workshop.

In any home workers scheme, the blind worker is provided with materials at home and makes a certain quota of goods which are later collected and marketed. Provided the blind person averages a certain minimum output per week, augmentation of wages is paid as in the workshops.

An example would be a blind person employed at home as a machine knitter; the knitting machine is provided by the local authority together with materials and orders. Each home worker so employed receives augmentation provided a certain agreed minimum productivity is maintained.

Blind persons are employed in similar occupations in home workers schemes as in the workshops. Although many blind home workers schemes are excellent, they do not provide such a satisfactory solution as workshop schemes. In particular, it is often difficult to supervise the blind people as satisfactorily and the blind persons themselves miss the company that they meet in a workshop. It is also more difficult for the blind person to concentrate on a high level of production—most homes contain too many distractions.

General social services for blind persons

(a) **Part-time occupations**. Some elderly blind people are keen to fill in a portion of their day by having a part-time occupation. This is usually arranged by the home teacher who helps organise any marketing assistance for articles produced. There are various arrangements to cope with this problem and many towns have a *disabled persons shop* which markets the products made in this way by blind or other disabled people.

Augmentation is never given to blind people working part-time as it is only intended to help and encourage those engaged in full-time work.

(b) **Learning to read**. An important part of any social service for the blind is concerned with home tuition in reading. There are two forms of embossed type:

1 *Moon*—raised letters—easy to learn but a very slow and inefficient method of reading which, for this reason, is not often taught.
2 *Braille*—this is the usual method of reading used by the blind. It is a complicated system of embossed dots arranged in a rectangular

pattern. It is taught to all blind children and younger blinded adults and elderly persons who have both the ability and desire to learn. It takes an intelligent blind person at least six months fairly hard study to learn Braille and, for this reason, is beyond the ability of many elderly persons who go blind in later life.

A useful indicator of the likelihood of an elderly person, who has recently developed blindness, learning Braille is given by finding out how much and what type of reading was undertaken before sight was lost. If the individual was an avid reader, it is always important to persevere with Braille. If, however, the blind person was a most casual reader of the simplest and widely illustrated newspapers, it is not likely that Braille will ever be learned.

All persons recently blinded under the age of about 50 years, and all young persons should always be taught Braille.

(c) Substitutes for reading. The Royal National Institute for the Blind have a large *library of recorded tapes of books read aloud*. They also lend a standard tape recorder to each blind and partially sighted person wishing to take advantage of this service. The person then borrows the tape recording of the required book, plays the tape and, in this way, can have a continuous and changing supply of books read aloud to him.

Each local authority makes a contribution to the Royal National Institute for the Blind for each person in its area who is using this service.

(d) Radios for the blind. The radio is a most useful service and greatly enjoyed by all blind people. There is a special voluntary society (Wireless for the Blind Fund) financed by the traditional appeal over the radio each Christmas Day, whose object is to ensure that every blind person is provided with a radio. Maintenance is arranged by local authorities.

(e) Special aids. Special aids in the home are available for the blind. A good example is the special braille form of 'regulo' which can be fitted to gas stoves to help the blind person who is cooking.

(f) Provision of guide-dogs for the blind. A society exists which provides and trains *special guide dogs* which can be used by the blind. The selection and training of the dog and blind person is lengthy and costly and necessarily limits the number of blind people who can be helped in this way. Only a few breeds are suitable for training, e.g. retrievers. In particular, it is a most valuable service for any active blind person living alone. Local authorities meet the cost of training and provision of guide-dogs which is, today, usually in the region of £2000.

(g) Holidays and hostels. The provision of *special holiday homes for the blind* is another general social function. Many of these are run by voluntary bodies, and local authorities assist by contributing and paying for the blind people from their area who use them. The holiday homes are specially adapted and make it possible for blind people to have a holiday on their own. The difficulties and dangers of going alone to ordinary hotels and boarding houses usually meant that blind people living alone did not take holidays.

There are a few specially designed permanent hostels for elderly blind people. But many more old people who are blind are looked after very satisfactorily in ordinary elderly persons hostels—perhaps two blind people in a hostel containing 40 sighted elderly persons—and in many ways the blind people seem to enjoy such hostels more.

(h) Financial help. Although local authorities cannot help blind people by direct money grants, there are *special pension facilities* available to blind people. It is the responsibility of the social workers employed by local authorities to make certain that the blind people understand what these are:

(a) for all blind persons aged 16 and over, the supplementary benefit scale rates are increased by £1.25 per week.

(b) there is a special £360 (single person) or £720 (married couple) income tax allowance for blind persons less any tax free disability payments.

(i) Voting. A blind person has a right to vote by post in parliamentary and local elections or to have his ballot paper marked with the help of a sighted person.

(j) Free postage. Free postage is allowed for a number of 'articles for the blind' including embossed literature, paper for embossing, and for recordings acting as an alternative to an embossed book.

(k) Television licence. There is a reduction of £1.25 in the cost of any television licence and the blind person does not need a dog licence for a guide dog.

Social services for other groups of disabled people

The social services described in detail above, provide a useful basis for a discussion of the services available to other handicapped persons.

In all groups, it is always important to arrange:

1   as complete a system of *registration* as possible
2   *individual assessment* by means of home visiting so that the difficulties

and problems of the handicapped person can be separately assessed in the surroundings of his own home.

Compared with the other social services described for blind people, there are many differences for other handicapped groups and these will now be discussed separately.

Deaf and dumb

This general term describes people who are *born completely deaf* and who, in the past, *never developed any speech*, not because of a defect of voice production, but because normal speech is only learnt by copying what is heard—a process impossible in the congenitally deaf. With very modern methods of teaching, it is now possible to teach speech to most congenitally deaf children.

The problems of the group as a whole are mainly connected with the isolation from which they suffer.

The need of most deaf and dumb people is, therefore, connected with arranging:

(a) suitable *interpreter services* in obtaining a job or in sorting out any difficulty; (b) *clubs and recreational facilities* for them. Many deaf and dumb people use a mixture of sign and finger language by which they converse with each other. Because of this, they enjoy mixing with other deaf and dumb people rather than normal people with whom they often find it difficult to communicate.

Lip reading is also used to understand speech and many deaf and dumb people find television very enjoyable.

Finding and keeping a suitable occupation is not usually a difficult problem for deaf and dumb people, provided they receive help, especially in interpretation from a trained social worker.

Most of the social services for deaf and dumb people are carried out by voluntary societies, many of whom are connected with church bodies. There is an historical reason for their welfare which was originally started in the nineteenth century by the church, with the object of providing special church services which deaf and dumb people could follow. Today welfare services have developed widely to include all types of social services, but there are still special religious services held weekly for deaf and dumb people in many places.

Hard of hearing

People who develop deafness, having in the past enjoyed good hearing, are usually referred to as '*hard of hearing*'. This term indicates that although deaf, such handicapped people have normal speech and listen either by lip reading or with the help of a hearing aid.

The greatest proportion of people who are hard of hearing are elderly, as deafness, like blindness, usually develops seriously in old age. It is important to make certain that:

(a) correct assessment of hearing is undertaken from time to time.

(b) that hearing aids are provided and are well maintained so that they are constantly helpful.

The assessment of hearing is usually carried out in an Ear, Nose and Throat department of a hospital, or in a special centre, such as those found in the school health service of large authorities. Hearing should always be tested by a pure tone audiometer. Coarse tests often used, such as listening to speech or the ticking of a watch, are of very limited value and of no use at all in assessing the degree of deafness to different frequencies of sound.

Probably there is no more neglected health aid than a hearing aid. The fitting of a hearing aid needs patience to ensure that it is fully understood by the deaf person, and is completely comfortable. Unless this is so and the deaf person understands its working, it is bound to be a failure. Care is also needed to maintain the aid and it is always helpful if a home visitor — health visitor or social worker—can call periodically on the deaf person to check that the aid is still in use and is satisfactory.

Paralytic conditions

This contains both progressive conditions (multiple sclerosis, muscular dystrophies) and non-progressive states—poliomyelitis and the sequelae of accidents.

Many of these individuals need a variety of community services outlined on pages 207–212. Occupation should be possible for those whose mobility is maintained and especially for mild cases. Much of the social help this group requires is assistance with housing, transport and the fitting of various aids to enable them to live more normal lives within the community.

Paraplegia

Many of these cases result from accidents in which the spinal cord is permanently injured. The extent of the paralysis will depend upon the site of the injury—the lower the site the better the outlook and vice versa. All will be paralysed from the waist down, but if this is the main lesion (i.e., if the arms are unaffected) then up to 80 per cent of patients should be able to lead reasonably normal lives and be able to follow an occupation.

Such disabled people can, with the aid of suitable mechanized transport, become quite mobile and they usually develop tremendous power in the arms to compensate and soon learn how to improvise.

Sporting facilities have always been an important part of social facilities provided for paraplegics. This is because the strengthening of compensatory muscles is an essential part of training those with paraplegia to overcome their disability. Following the lead given by Stoke Mandeville Hospital both national and international sporting events are held each year culminating in the Paraplegic Olympics which are held in the same year as the Olympic Games. Many different sporting activities are suitable including archery, basket ball, etc. Some local authorities assist paraplegics by providing suitable premises and sports centres where these activities can take place.

Cerebral palsy

Many spastic handicapped people need similar services to those with other paralytic or crippling diseases. Most of these conditions date from birth and, therefore, suitable education and training facilities for the young adolescent are important. Speech defects also pose special difficulties.

Recent work has emphasized that it is better to look after spastics in conjunction with other handicapped people. About 25 per cent of spastics also suffer from epilepsy and, therefore, for this group the services outlined below may also be important.

Epilepsy

People with epilepsy present many problems not met with in other groups of handicapped people. This is not due to the unusual difficulties of treating epilepsy, but to the ill-informed and unfair attitude of the public generally.

Most people with epilepsy suffer from minor degrees of the illness and are well controlled and can quite satisfactorily be employed in most professions and occupations. In fact, there are many examples of people who have mild epilepsy, succeeding in most occupations. But the public have an unreasonable fear of people with this disease because quite wrongly they assume that the person with epilepsy may be dangerous. Some people even think the disease is some form of mental illness. All this adverse public reaction leads to many patients with epilepsy concealing the fact that they have had occasional epileptic seizures, because they fear if it is known they have epilepsy, they may lose their jobs or find it difficult to find employment. The strain of concealing these facts is considerable, especially as a sudden unexpected attack of epilepsy at work, could, at any time, lead to discovery. For this reason, many patients in good posts live in constant fear of discovery and this often leads to the development of other difficulties including a minor anxiety state.

To help the person with epilepsy, it is important to realize this difficult background and to try and arrange for the employer or prospective employer to know the full facts and that his epilepsy, if properly controlled, may be no hazard. It is usual for those with epilepsy to have some form of warning of an impending attack and, apart from avoiding a few dangerous occupations in which he will rarely want to work, there are few jobs which are not suitable.

It is, however, essential that a constant and careful watch is kept on each person with epilepsy to make sure that the treatment received is controlling the disease.

The final success of any treatment depends on complete rehabilitation. Because of this, it is most helpful to attach a specially trained health visitor or social worker to the hospital which treats most serious epilepsy, so that all the social aspects of the illness—home, occupation, etc.—can be carefully investigated. In this way, much preventive work can be done and many problems can be avoided or corrected before they can have a serious effect.

Occasionally, it is necessary to admit to an epileptic colony a person whose epilepsy is uncontrollable or whose home is quite unsuitable. Most epileptic colonies are run by voluntary bodies and local authorities meet the cost. Although most people in colonies have to stay there permanently, every effort is made to rehabilitate them sufficiently to return to community life if at all possible.

Special medical assessment and treatment centres for epilepsy.

Important special centres for medical assessment of difficult cases of epilepsy have been set up for children at Oxford (based on the Park Hospital for Children) and for adults at York and Chalfont (Bucks). Skilled assessment in difficult cases is essential and such units are just beginning to probe some of the complicated facets of some cases of epilepsy.

15
Care of Mentally Disordered People

Role of local authorities

The social services departments of local authorities are responsible for developing widespread community social services for the mentally disordered (mentally ill and mentally handicapped). These fall mainly, into three categories:

1 Social work support provided by social workers (formerly called mental welfare officers).
2 Day care facilities to help with the reintegration of anyone who has had mental illness or is mentally handicapped. These include social rehabilitation, occupational therapy, industrial therapy and workshop provision.
3 Residential facilities for those who have no satisfactory home to return to after their illness.

Law relating to the mentally disordered

Major changes in the law concerning mentally disordered persons were made in 1959 and again in 1982, subsequently being consolidated into a single Act in 1983:

Mental Health Act 1959

The Mental Health Act, 1959, changed the entire law relating to all forms of mental illness and handicap. This followed the realization that a completely new approach was essential if progress was to be made in the prevention and care of mental illness and handicap.

There were 4 main aims in the Mental Health Act of 1959 which are still central to the 1983 Act:

1 To remove wherever possible the stigma attached to mental illness.
2 To bring mental illness and mental handicap under the same code of practice.
3 To bring the medical treatment of mental illness and mental handicap on to the same basis as the treatment of physical illness.

4   To develop as far as possible community social services for the mentally ill and handicapped.

(1) *The removal of stigma* attached to mental illness is not easy as it is necessary to change the attitude of public opinion to mental disability. Due to ignorance as to its cause, many people feel ashamed, or have feelings of guilt, when a member of their family develops some form of mental illness.

There is really no basis at all for such a reaction. Hardly any mental illness is hereditary. Mental illness is not uncommon—each year 439 per 100 000 of the population are admitted to mental hospitals in England and one third of these are admitted for the first time.

It has been estimated that one in 20 to 25 people are admitted to a mental hospital at some time in their life while probably double that number seek advice from their family doctor for an illness whose basis is primarily mental not physical. This means that few, if any families, do not contain some member who has had or will have some form of mental illness.

Probably one of the most effective ways to help reduce stigma would be for all large district general hospitals to have mental health departments which would replace the isolated mental hospitals. This would mean that the reason for a patient's admission would not be so obvious—as it is when admitted to a mental hospital. It would also help to improve understanding between doctors and nurses treating physical and mental illnesses.

(2) Until 1959, *mental illness*, that is a disease whose main problem is some form of *emotional instability*, was treated quite separately, in the legal as well as medical sense, from *mental handicap*, which is primarily a defect of development of the intellect in which *the intelligence of the patient is seriously retarded.* From the pathological aspect, it is reasonable to consider them separately. However, in the individual case both factors often play a part. For example, in a case of mental handicap (in which the intelligence of the person is retarded) the prognosis will depend, to some extent, on the person's emotional stability. If this is quite normal, there is much more chance of successfully training him to carry out some occupation and lead a reasonably normal life. However, if there is even a moderate degree of emotional instability, this may prove impossible.

From 1959 the Law has dealt with both forms of mental disability— *mental illness* and *mental handicap.*

(3) *Treatment of physical illness* is designed to carry out a full investigation, to correct various pathological processes discovered and, if possible, to restore the patient to full health. If this is not possible, the aim is to arrest development of the disease and to control problems. Treatment may take place at home by the family doctor, or the patient may be referred to hospital either as an out-patient or an in-patient for investigation and treatment. But once these are completed, the patient invariably returns home. Even in the case of a steadily developing disease

with a fatal outlook, such as a malignant new growth, the patient is sent home and remains there as long as possible.

The *treatment of all forms of mental disability* has the following important differences:

(a) There is usually a question of protecting both the patient and the community from the effects of the mental illness—e.g., the danger of suicide (a special problem is endogenous depression or if there is any insomnia in puerperal depression—immediately after birth—for such symptoms may be seen in women just before a serious suicide attempt). Occasionally violent behaviour is noted (even criminal behaviour) which means that special arrangements have to be made to admit a few patients compulsorily and to retain them by compulsion in a mental hospital (*custodial care*).

(b) Much mental illness and handicap is a long standing or chronic problem whereas the majority of physical hospital patients are acute or sub-acute patients who are being treated for a short time.

Because the cause of illness for mentally ill or handicapped people compared with physical illness was so little understood until recently few effective and dramatic treatments were available to them.

Fifty years ago, mental hospitals were almost entirely asylums—places where the immates could safely be cared for rather than treated. Because of this, many who entered them remained there as in-patients for may years, and often for the rest of their lives.

New treatments, electrical convulsion therapy, leucotomy, the introduction of many tranquillizer drugs, better rehabilitation facilities and social services have changed all this. This aim today is to use hospital admission in mental disability mainly for investigation and early treatment, and then to return the individual home for follow-up treatment and special social services after-care and rehabilitation. Occasionally it is still necessary to arrange an admission compulsorily, but it is hoped this will eventually occur only rarely. Wherever possible, the patient is encouraged to be admitted as a *voluntary patient* even if acutely mentally ill.

(4) *The development of widespread community social services* has made it possible for continuing treatment to be carried out while the person lives at home. If home conditions are not suitable, the individual may live in a *special hostel* provided by the social services department or by a voluntary organization. Such an arrangement is more normal and therefore to be preferred. Occasionally *boarding out* may be arranged with sympathetic persons who understand mental disability. Another excellent arrangement is to provide sheltered flats where two mentally handicapped people can live together quite independently.

Successful community care will only be possible if a wide range of supporting social services are available—social workers skilled in after-care work, *hostels, adult training centres, special workshops, occupational therapy, clubs, job placement services* leading, if possible, to full-time employment being obtained in ordinary industry.

Such extended social services (provided by social services departments) must be supported by better training of general practitioners and home nurses in the medical care of the chronic mentally disordered individual. Both the community social services (provided by social workers) and the community health services (general practitioners, home nurses, community psychiatric nurses, health visitors) must work very closely together so that all complement each other.

Reform of Mental Health Legislation—Mental Health (Amendment) Act 1982, now consolidated into the Mental Health Act 1983

Reform of certain parts of the Mental Health Act, 1959, was mainly directed to increasing the safeguards for patients' rights.

The Mental Health (Amendment) Act 1982 became law in late 1982 and its main changes included:

1 *Definitions.* The terms *mental impairment* and *severe mental impairment* replace 'mental subnormality' and 'severe mental subnormality' (see pp. 234–5). Alcoholism, drug dependency and sexual deviancy are specifically excluded as not being part of the definition of mental disorder.

2 *Compulsory Admission procedures.* The powers of s. 4, s. 2, and s. 3 (replacing s. 29, s. 25 and s. 26 of the 1959 Act) were modified in the following ways:

Section 4 Mental Health Act 1983—Emergency admissions. (Replacing Section 29 of the Mental Health Act 1959). In future:

(a) the applicant must examine the patient within 24 hours of making the application (rather than within 3 days as at present);

(b) only the *patient's nearest relative* (not any relative as at present) or an *approved social worker* will be allowed to make the application;

(c) admission will have to be carried out within 24 hours of the medical examination or the application (rather than within 3 days).

Section 2 Mental Health Act 1983—Admission for observation for 28 days. (Replacing Section 25 of Mental Health Act 1959). In future:

(a) s. 2 to be used for the purpose of *assessment* rather than observation;

(b) the patient will have power to appeal against detention to a Mental Health Review Tribunal within the first 14 days of detention;

(c) the nearest relative will be given a discharge power.

Section 3 Mental Health Act 1983 – Admission for one year's treatment with periods of renewal. (Replacing Section 26 of the Mental Health Act 1959). The longer term power of detention under s. 3 has been amended to remove age limits and to include a treatability test. This applies only to *mental handicap and psychopathic disorder* and ensures that only patients who can benefit from treatment will be able to be compulsorily detained in hospital.

3 *Qualifications of the social worker.* The Act provides for the role now being undertaken by mental welfare officers to be taken over after November 1984 by approved social workers who will have to interview any patient prior to their compulsory admission to hospital, to ensure that this is the most appropriate form of care.

Regulations have been introduced defining the training of approved social workers. This change is designed to meet the criticism that, since 1971, there has been a lack of specialisation in social workers responsible for compulsory admissions.

4 *Consent to treatment.* This clause proposes that:

(a) treatments that give rise to special concern (i.e. those which might be hazardous, irreversible or not fully established) will in future require the patient's consent *and* agreement of an independent doctor;

(b) other treatments, including surgical treatment, administration of medicine and electroconvulsive therapy, which do not give rise to special concern may be given with the patient's consent or without it, if a second opinion agrees;

(c) all other care, attention and treatment can be given without the patient's consent;

(d) in certain circumstances, treatments can be given in an emergency without reference to the above procedures.

5 *Mental Health Act Commission.* This Commission was proposed by the Amendment Act 1982 and set up in September 1983. Its main responsibilities include:

(a) the exercise of general protective functions for detained patients;

(b) the visiting and interviewing of detained patients;

(c) ensuring that patients are informed of their rights;

(d) examining the lawfulness of detention;

(e) investigating complaints.

6 *Extending the opportunities for patients to have their cases considered by Mental Health Review Tribunals.* Seven changes are introduced including:

(a) increasing the opportunities for patients to apply to tribunals by halving detention periods;

(b) automatic referrals to tribunals for patients who do not exercise their right of application in the first 6 months or who have not been reviewed by a tribunal for 3 years;

(c) a right of application to a tribunal for patients detained under s. 2 of the Mental Health Act 1983;

(d) providing the tribunals with power to order a delayed discharge;

(e) permitting a patient to withdraw an application to a tribunal without losing his right of application;

(f) changes in the criteria which the tribunal must consider in reviewing a patient's case;

(g) allowing children under the age of 16 years to apply for a tribunal on their own behalf and to initiate automatic referrals for children who have not been reviewed for one year.

The Mental Health Act 1983

This Act became Law in October 1983. It consolidates the Mental Health Act 1959 (see page 224) and the Mental Health (Amendment) Act 1982 (see page 227) into a single piece of legislation. Some of the Section numbers have been changed. All those given here are the 1983 Act numbers with their original equivalents in brackets, where appropriate.

Generally the changes in the Mental Health Act 1983 have been welcomed although certain bodies including MIND have indicated that they would have liked to see wider powers introduced to ensure that mental health legislation should not be considered principally with the exercise of compulsory powers and attendant safeguards but with the creation of a comprehensive legal framework for treatment and care mainly within a normal community environment. Concern has also been voiced that the Act fails to take initiatives to meet the needs and to safeguard the rights of informal patients.

The mentally ill

It is convenient to discuss social services for the mentally ill first under the following headings:

1 prevention
2 housing
3 hostels
4 occupation
5 general after-care
6 day care
7 hospital admissions

(1) Prevention of mental illness

Much preventive work in the mental health field is concerned *with the avoidance of further breakdown*, rather than with the initial mental illness.

In many instances, however, the extrinsic factors (see page 141) connected with the patient's environment especially at certain times of life, puberty, pregnancy, menopause, old age, are the precipitating cause of the start of the mental illness or a further breakdown.

Because of the extreme importance of the early years of life on the subsequent development of any person, it is *most important to recognize early, if possible, unusual signs of insecurity in a child*, as this is likely to indicate unsatisfactory home conditions. Most maternity and child health services today have a close link with a child psychiatrist and psychiatric social worker so that health visitors may discuss such cases and get help with their preventive work.

Social work support should be available to such a home at any time and the decision about who is best fitted to provide this should be made after joint discussion between doctors, health visitors, community psychiatric nurses and social workers.

In the same way, close liaison should always be maintained between child guidance staff who are helping schoolchildren with emotional or behavioural disorders and social workers who may have to provide after-care later.

(2) Housing

Housing conditions which are unsatisfactory for the mental development of a child may be quite different from those precipitating physical illness. The home may be very well provided with the physical essentials of life, but the *important mental factor of stability, love and affection may be missing.* Some of the worst environments are those homes in which parental strife is continuous and unending, perhaps eventually leading to separation of divorce. For this reason, particular attention must always be paid by the health visitor or the social worker to any home with such a background.

Even when early recognition of mental health problems has been made, it is never easy to change that home so that it becomes satisfactory. But, it is always a great help to know the problem exists and it is usually possible to prevent the effects of the poor home conditions being very detrimental to the child.

The value of the right type of home is just as important for the person who has had a mental illness and has been successfully treated in hospital. It may be much better for such a person to go to a special hostel on discharge from hospital rather than return to an unsuitable home.

(3) Hostels (small homes)

Hostels can be of various types and are provided by either the social services department or by a voluntary body. The aim should always be to achieve maximum integration between those living in them and the ordinary community. This is easier if the hostels are small, accommodating 6–8 persons and if they are scattered throughout the area rather than built together. As far as possible, hostels should be like ordinary houses; they can be established successfully in the older larger house or by modifying 2–3 adjacent terraced houses together on a modern council estate. *Boarding out* can also be useful as an alternative to an unsuitable home provided sympathetic and understanding hosts can be found. Because of this difficulty few successful boarding out schemes have yet been introduced by local authorities.

(4) Occupation

A carefully chosen occupation can do much to prevent a person developing a mental illness or to avoid a relapse, and is always an important factor in rehabilitation.

Many large industrial firms and HM Forces carefully examine all new entrants to assess as far as possible the type of personality, intelligence, aptitude and emotional stability, so that the person can be fitted into the most suitable occupation. This is most valuable and forms an important part of any occupational health service, for correct selection of occupation can avoid many breakdowns.

Having fitted the new entrant into his job, it is equally important that a careful watch is kept on him in the early period of his employment so that any signs of undue strain are recognized. This is also a valuable part of all *student health services* at Universities for it is known that serious mental illness can be avoided in students by ensuring early recognition of signs of stress.

It is the duty of a specially trained officer of the Employment Services Division, called a *Disablement Resettlement Officer* (DRO) (see page 208), to find employment for all handicapped people including those who are mentally disabled. It is often difficult to find employment for persons who have had a mental illness. They may have lost their original job and there is usually a resistance among employers to re-employ them for fear they will again break down and perhaps dislocate their staff.

Because of these problems it is most important that any unavoidable delay should not depress the person who has just left a mental hospital. *Occupational therapy at a special rehabilitation centre* or attendance at a day centre should always be provided as this will not only help in training him in physical skills (see below) but what is probably most important, it will do much to restore his self-confidence and get him used to meeting other people at the centre and prepare him for normal working conditions.

Social workers assist the Disablement Resettlement Officer in trying to find suitable jobs for those recovering from mental illnesses. Some social services departments have found it useful to employ a full-time officer to do this task. Much of this work is slow, and in one year such an officer may only find employment for a few patients. His efforts, however, not only in finding jobs for those who otherwise would probably have been unemployed, but by meeting employers, are constantly helping to educate the public in the problems of mental illness. The successful placement of one such person very often leads to another post being found in the same firm.

(5) General after-care

Follow-up after-care work is always most important as most who have had a mental illness will need long-term help. Much of this will be done by the person's own family doctor. However, much after-care is carried out by *social workers* from the social services department working closely with the family doctor.

All social aspects—home, family, occupation, etc., play an important part in after-care and the social worker must ensure that close co-operation exists so that the person who has recovered from a mental breakdown is given every opportunity to return to normal life as quickly as possible.

(6) Day Care Facilities for the mentally ill

Day care facilities play an increasingly important role in the rehabilitation of many former mental hospital patients. Such centres should provide a wide opportunity for the individual to meet many different people and to improve their social rehabilitation. Many such people lack confidence and their self-respect has been shaken by their illness. They need to gain confidence by demonstrating that they can manage quite well on their own (when they are away from their families). Daily attendance at such centres which are reached by a bus or train journey helps them greatly to gain such self-confidence.

The functions of such centres often overlap those of day hospitals and sheltered employment. *Occupational therapy* should be available at day centres. As well as helping with the problems of readjusting to the demands of work, *cultural and educational activities* such as a study of art, music, drama or literature should also be provided at day centres. As regards the organization of such centres, those attending them should be encouraged to help in their daily running.

(7) Hospital admission

Most hospital admissions for mental illness today are arranged in the same way as in physical illness—by the family doctor arranging for the patient to go into hospital as a voluntary patient. Approximately 85 per cent of all admissions are informal or voluntary. The decision is made after discussion between the family doctor and the psychiatrist who will then treat the patient in hospital.

Occasionally it is necessary to arrange *compulsory admission* and detention in hospital of a mentally ill patient for observation or as an urgent necessity.

In the admission for observation, application must be made by the patient's relative or the social worker of the local authority. This must be accompanied by written recommendations of two medical practitioners; one of these doctors must be specially approved under the Mental Health Act, 1983 Section 2 (see page 227).

In an emergency, compulsory admission can be arranged by application of a patient's relative or the social worker of the local authority, plus one written recommendation of a doctor. In this case detention only lasts 72 hours unless a second medical opinion is received (Section 4, Mental Health Act, 1983, see page 227).

Mental health review tribunals

There are many safeguards to make certain that no patient is retained in hospital compulsorily unless it is essential. Special *Mental Health Review Tribunals* are set up in each area to deal with any requests from patients for discharge.

After hearing the application the tribunal may direct the patient's discharge. It must do so if it is satisfied:

(a) that he is no longer suffering from mental illness, psychopathic disorder, subnormality or severe subnormality

(b) that it is not in the interests of the patient's health or safety or for the protection of other persons, that the patient should continue to be detained

(c) in the case of a psychopathic or subnormal patient whose discharge at the age of 25 was barred or a patient whose discharge by his nearest relative was barred, that if released he would not be likely to act in a manner dangerous to others or himself.

Note that under the Mental Health Act 1983 there is increased opportunity for mental patients to have their cases considered by the Mental Health Review Tribunal (see p. 228).

Mentally Handicapped People

Definitions

Mental handicap is a colloquial term in general use. It is not a legal term. The Mental Health Act 1983 introduces two new terms 'severe mental impairment' and 'mental impairment'. Both are similar but vary in degree. 'Mental impairment' is defined as a state of arrested or incomplete development of the mind which includes significant impairment of intelligence and social functioning *and is associated with abnormally aggressive or seriously irresponsible conduct.*

Note that all people who are mentally impaired are also mentally handicapped but that only a proportion of mentally handicapped people are also mentally impaired. Mental impairment is a legal term and people with this disability are liable to various actions under the Mental Health Act 1983. The terms 'severe mental impairment' and 'mental impairment' in the Mental Health Act 1983 have replaced the terms 'severe mental subnormality' and 'mental subnormality' which should no longer be used.

There is a tendency to classify mentally handicapped people only according to their intellectual level, by means of intelligence tests (see page 83). However, it is well known that intelligence tests often give unreliable results in people with such handicap. The tests take no account of the individual as a whole—his personality, behaviour and skills—and the results can vary according to the motivation of the person being tested and the particular test used.

The basis for determining whether or not someone is mentally handicapped and what degree of handicap they have therefore depends on:

1   An estimate of their intelligence.
2   A social test to judge the ability of the individual to make use of his intelligence (i.e. a test of performance). Generally children who are three years or more behind their average age group in school are probably mentally handicapped, unless there is another cause for their learning difficulties (e.g. deafness or prolonged absence from formal classwork because of physical illness).
3   The emotional stability of the person. The majority of those who are mentally handicapped need special help from social services.

The range of mental handicap is wide. Some people are said to be in the 'borderline group'. Their intellect is very nearly what is considered normal, and they may have an IQ of between 70 and 85. Although they may have had a deprived background, difficulties at school and in finding employment ultimately they integrate well with society and do not need help from the social services. Handicapped people who are only able to lead an independent life if given special support, in care and training are sometimes said to be mildly or moderately handicapped. Their IQ is usually below about 65. People with profound mental handicap (IQ below about 45) are unable to lead an independent life or to guard themselves against exploitation. They are sometimes said to have 'special needs' or to require 'special care'. They are usually multiply handicapped and require nursing and physiotherapy; they often have a reduced lifespan.

Incidence of mental handicap

In England, approximately 38 000 mentally handicapped people of all ages are receiving day care services from local authority social services departments. About 48 000 severely mentally handicapped people are looked after in hospitals but this number is steadily diminishing as emphasis is laid on looking after as many as possible in the community.

Causes of mental handicap

Most mental handicap is present at birth and generally results from a mutation in which the individual is left with an incomplete development of the mind. Mentally handicapped people may belong to a recognized type such as Down's syndrome (previously called mongolism because of the characteristic facial development reminiscent of Mongol races) which is known to be caused by a chromosome abnormality.

Occasionally mental handicap may follow severe birth injury—thus approximately 48 per cent of those with cerebral palsy have some degree of mental handicap. Although there is a relationship between the degree of spasticity and intelligence quotient, it is important to realize that this is not invariable *for a few very severely spastic individuals have normal intelligence quotients.*

Reference has already been made to that rare metabolic disease— phenylketonuria (see page 60)—in which the child is born almost normal but soon his defective metabolism leads to a poisoning of the brain which results in developmental delay within a few months. If phenylketonuria is diagnosed early—within six weeks of birth, and the child is fed on a special diet, there is every hope that the development will be normal. It is for this reason that the blood of all babies is tested by the midwife and health visitor on the tenth day and between four and six weeks of life to make certain that every case is discovered (more details about this test on page 60). It is equally important to recognize hypothyroidism by screening babies by a blood test (see page 60).

Mental handicap occasionally develops following a *severe infection of the brain or meninges.* For this reason, it is *essential that no delay ever occurs in diagnosing and treating such conditions.*

Prevention of mental handicap

The opportunities to prevent handicap are increasing rapidly. The following is a list of likely ways to avoid it.

1 **Genetic counselling.** The aim in genetic counselling is to identify where there is a high risk of the transmission of hereditary disease leading to mental handicap. At present this is usually only possible after the birth of one affected child (unless there is a family history as in Huntington's chorea). In some cases it may be possible to estimate the risks of another handicapped child being born. If these are high because one parent is a carrier of an abnormality which is likely to show itself in other children, then the parents can seek family planning help to prevent conception of another child.

    With modern techniques it is possible to predict the chances of parents who have already had one Down's syndrome child having another. In the majority of instances the risks are small, but in a few cases the risk is high and these are the families in which genetic counselling can help.

2 **Amniocentesis** (removal of a small quantity of amniotic fluid). Chromosome abnormalities can be detected at 16 weeks, in time to enable a termination of pregnancy to be carried out if investigations show that the fetus is abnormal. This is advised routinely for pregnant women aged 38 and over and for anyone who has already had a Down's syndrome baby (see also p. 43).

3 **Immunization of girls against rubella.** Immunization between the ages of 11–14 years will prevent rubella infection which in the first three months of pregnancy may lead to brain damage in the foetus.

4 **Use of anti-D-immunoglobulin** to prevent haemolytic disease of new born (see pages 40–41).

5 **Expert care in labour** to reduce the risk of hypoxia and brain damage to the infant.

6 **Intensive care during neonatal period** for babies of low birth weight.

7 **Screening to prevent phenylketonuria** (see page 60) and other metabolic diseases.

8 **Earlier completion of families** will reduce the chance of a mentally

handicapped child being born. The effect of this is shown by the increased chances of a Down's syndrome child being born to the older woman.

Social services for mentally handicapped people

Importance of co-ordination and a multidisciplinary approach

Although this section mainly describes social services, it is essential to realize that the *medical, educational, psychological and social needs* should be considered together. No single profession can tackle successfully all the problems and the use of an *assessment team* is important.

In young children the paediatrician, psychiatrist, child psychologist, health visitor, social worker and educationalist will all be involved as well as the family doctor.

Table 15.1 Incidence of Down's syndrome, Sweden 1968–70 (331 000 births)

Age of mother	Incidence
−19	1 in 1695 births
20–24	1 in 1351 births
25–29	1 in 1136 births
30–34	1 in 685 births
35–39	1 in 267 births
40–44	1 in 67 births
45 +	1 in 16 births

(from Lindsjo (1974) *Acta Paediatr. Scand* **63** 571/516)

Older children will need educational, social and vocational assessment. Adults may require repeated assessments from psychiatrists, clinical psychologist, general practitioners and social workers. Much of this assessment will take place in hospitals, schools, training centres, workshops or in the individual's own home.

Community social services

Many of the main social services of local authorities aim to provide a supportive community service in which the mentally handicapped persons and their families are encouraged to live a more normal life. If possible such individuals should be trained to follow a full-time occupation.

Since the introduction of the Education (Handicapped Children) Act, 1971, the care of mentally handicapped children up to the age of 19 years has been transferred to the education services (see page 82).

Many varied types of assistance are provided by social services departments of local authorities including:

1 Social work support or counselling
2 Practical help—home help, day nurseries, laundry services, sitters-in, etc.
3 Training and day centres for adults
4 Occupational therapy centres
5 Workshops for adults
6 Employment in ordinary industry
7 Small homes (hostels)
8 Short-term or respite care
9 Holidays and recreational activities—clubs, etc.

(1) Social work support and counselling

Parents need much help to adjust to the problems of caring for a mentally handicapped child. Many professionals are involved—doctors, health visitors, teachers and social workers. Much of the domiciliary visiting in the community is undertaken by social workers especially after initial diagnosis and assessment.

Although education authorities are now responsible for the education of mentally handicapped children in special schools, much of the social work for this group, e.g. visiting at home, is carried out by social workers from the social services department. This has the great advantage of improving co-ordination between the education and social services departments and enabling continuity of care to be maintained when the child reaches the age of 19, ends formal education and then comes under the direct supervision of the social services department.

(2) Practical help

Many families facing the problems of caring for a mentally handicapped individual may need the assistance of *home helps* (see page 266), *day nurseries* (see page 181), *laundry services. Sitters-in* can be of great help to enable the parents to get a short break.

(3) Training centres for adults

Adult training centres or social education centres are provided by social service departments and designed to carry on the training of mentally handicapped people who have left special school. Many are mixed but some are single sex centres. The main task of the centre is to concentrate on training mentally handicapped people in some skill, preferably within ordinary employment. A few adult mentally handicapped people may find it difficult to adjust themselves to such training, but with the modern workshop whose tasks are more diverse, these should be exceptions (see p. 240).

Social training should continue in the adult training centres and all should concentrate on mastering the skills of helping run a home and becoming more skilled in various hobbies and pastimes. It is very often in these training sessions that a simple concept of numbers is understood.

It is most important to recognize the *importance of inducement and constant encouragement*. The mentally handicapped individual *must* be given targets to achieve and not just left to work at his own pace. The *potential of many mentally handicapped people is far higher than expected*, but full potential will only be reached by training which constantly pushes each individual to his fullest capacity.

(4) Family therapy

Training given in a centre should always be linked with home life so that handicapped people enjoy participating domestically. The handicapped person's family, too, may need continuing, though not necessarily constant support. They should be encouraged to include their handicapped member in all their activities since stimulation and a loving and secure environment, as with all children, will help development. In addition to home visits by professionals informal family group meetings allow ideas to be exchanged, problems to be aired and are also social occasions.

Problems occasionally arise as puberty develops in these mentally handicapped people. It should always be carefully explained to parents that close supervision must be maintained on the activities of their child at home. In particular, it is most important that *every parent of a mentally handicapped girl realizes that her mental handicap will make her more vulnerable to the advances of unscrupulous men.*

(5) Occupational therapy centres

Some occupational therapy centres are also used to help mentally handicapped people. At such centres occupational therapists give mentally handicapped individuals an opportunity to become involved in many different activities. These include various handicrafts and also training in group activities. If possible evening clubs should be arranged and run in such a way that the mentally handicapped people themselves do much of the organization (see also Section 10 on page 242).

(6) Workshops

There has been widespread development during the last few years in the setting up of a *sheltered workshop* within an adult training centre by local authorities, in which mentally handicapped adults are employed.

The types of workshops vary greatly, but include:

(i) carrying out simple tasks, which can only be undertaken by hand; occasionally these are contracted out to the workshops by industry and undertaken by mentally handicapped people. Such tasks vary but in one group of workshops include:

(a) fixing a pourer into the top of a salt container
(b) stamping tight the top of another container
(c) assembling packs of picnic cups
(d) assembling ball-point pens

(ii) manufacturing 'own products' such as the making of wooden and soft toys or furniture which are then sold locally.

Because of the necessity to fit the regime into that of industry, the workshop remains open for the whole of the year. Although the workshop is, in effect, a place of employment for many mentally handicapped people, the training processes still continue. This is often seen in the method of payment adopted. One successful scheme is to base weekly payment upon a 'points' system, by which points, which represent part of the maximum wage, are added for good steady work and rate and standard of production, and deducted for bad behaviour, lateness or non-attendance. In this way the mentally handicapped people employed at the workshop quickly learn the importance of hard work and good behaviour.

Inducement is an essential part of workshop training and the method of financial remuneration used should encourage better productivity, hardwork and better social behaviour.

It is usual to arrange that the maximum 'wage' be equal to the maximum amount each may earn without having any deduction made from his supplementary benefit. At present, this means each mentally subnormal person employed at the workshops may earn £4 per week without any deduction being made in his supplementary benefit.

One of the most encouraging and remarkable changes which has always been reported following the successful introduction of workshops for mentally handicapped persons has been the great improvement in the behaviour and outlook of those working in them. Almost without exception, they become better behaved, easier to control and seem to be very delighted to realize that at last they are 'earning'—they obviously feel they have made a great step forward by having shown they can do a useful occupation. There is little doubt that the introduction of such workshops has done much to improve the opportunities and facilities for the adult mentally handicapped person.

(7) Employment in open industry

Until very recently few opportunities occurred for mentally handicapped people to move on from workshops to working in ordinary industry. Successful workshops report that it is possible to find work in ordinary industry for at least 10 per cent of the mentally handicapped who have been trained in the workshops. The success of this must depend to some extent on the employment opportunities in the district and the present high level of unemployment is making it very difficult. It is, however, *most important that all those working with mentally handicapped people* realize their potential *which in a substantial minority includes successful employment in ordinary industry.*

(8) Small homes (hostels)

Most social services departments now provide special homes where mentally handicapped persons can live when for any reason they have to leave home. In some cases there is a need to provide a hostel (home) where the mentally handicapped person can live during his rehabilitation after discharge from hospital. It is most important that no-one is ever kept in hospital any longer than is absolutely necessary, otherwise they become institutionalised and further rehabilitation is very difficult.

The term 'home' is often used instead of 'hostel' because it is hoped that it will not give the impression of impermanence or of a certain austerity. All should provide a homely atmosphere and be friendly. The purpose of the home should be to provide a permanent substitute family home.

The size of each home varies, but it should not exceed 20 and many excellent ones are much smaller containing 4 to 5 individuals.

It is important that all mentally handicapped persons living in the home partake of ordinary duties just as if they were living with their own family. These include the cooking of breakfast and the preparation of a light evening meal.

Every effort should be made to integrate these homes completely within the community—children should attend normal special schools (i.e. not a school solely for the residents), adults should go out to work either in ordinary industry or in special workshops. The activities of the residents should be as nearly the same as those people in a normal home environment.

(9) Short-term or 'respite' care

Very many mentally handicapped children are looked after in their own homes by devoted parents. There is, however, a great deal of strain involved and many parents find the continuous caring process produces considerable problems for the family.

It is important that the devotion of such parents is not continued in such a way that matrimonial difficulties occur, and that other normal members of the family are not neglected.

One of the most useful aids in preventing this danger is for social services departments to provide '*short-term*' *care* in which special temporary arrangements are made to look after the mentally handicapped child for a short period (two to three weeks to enable the parents and family to get a complete break. It has been found that such short-term care helps such parents considerably and enables them to return refreshed to the arduous task of looking after a severely handicapped child.

It is also important to provide some shorter breaks for parents by arranging for experienced 'sitters in' who can look after the mentally handicapped child while the parents have an evening out. In some instances, it helps to arrange residential care for one night or a weekend.

(10) Holidays, recreational activities (social centres, clubs, etc.)

Most social service departments provide social centres or clubs for mentally handicapped people where they can pursue pastimes and form a *club*. Such activities are valuable in helping them to gain confidence, to enjoy themselves and to get used to meeting people. Social workers often attend such centres and, in this way, keep in touch with their clients.

Holidays of various kinds are also arranged. Some of these are traditional type holidays but others are of a more ambitious type (i.e. adventure type of holidays, camping, etc.).

Services provided by hospitals for mentally handicapped people

A certain proportion of profoundly mentally handicapped adults are unable to settle at home or in a training centre, and it may be necessary to admit them to a special hospital. A few will always have to remain there because of their inability to learn even simple social habits, or because of extreme mental instability and behavioural problems. It is always the aim of the authorities to rehabilitate people to such a degree that they can be discharged to attend adult training centres. Close co-ordination is always maintained between the staff of the hospital and the staff of the domiciliary mental handicap service. It is generally agreed that everything should be done to ensure that no mentally handicapped child or adult ever remains permanently in hospital.

Special legal powers for mentally disordered people

Criminal proceedings

In criminal proceedings, courts have power to authorize the admission and detention of a mentally disordered person found guilty of offences by the Courts. A *Hospital Order* may be made if the court is satisfied that, on the written or oral evidence of two doctors (one of whom must be specially approved), the offender is suffering from mental illness, severe mental impairment, mental impairment or psychopathic disorder warranting hospital treatment. This order authorizes the removal of a patient to hospital within 28 days. The Court may, if necessary, make an order for the detention of the patient in a *place of safety*, which includes residential accommodation provided by a Local Authority, a hospital or mental nursing home, a residential home for mentally disordered persons, a police station or any other suitable place where the occupier is willing to receive the patient.

Alternatively the Court may make a *Guardianship Order* instead of a Hospital Order if it is thought that the client should be cared for within the community. It is usual in such cases for local authorities to assume the office of Guardianship.

Protection and management of property and affairs

Any person who becomes mentally incapable of managing his own affairs, cannot legally authorize anyone else to do this on his behalf. If power of attorney has been given to another person before the mental illness then such authority will probably become inoperable because of the illness. In such cases, the *Court of Protection* exists to protect and manage the affairs and property of any person who is mentally incapable of doing so. The Court of Protection usually appoints a *receiver*—usually a close relative (parent, brother or sister)—to administer the patient's affairs under the direction of the Court. This will continue until the Court of Protection is satisfied on medical evidence that the patient is now fit again.

Application to the Court of Protection (at 25 Store Street, London WC1) can be made by a close relative or by instructing a solicitor to make such an approach.

16
Care of the Elderly

Proportion of elderly within the community

The proportion of old people in our community has been steadily rising during the last seventy years. At the start of the twentieth century, about 5 per cent of the population were of retirement age. Today, in the United Kingdom, 16 per cent are of retirement age (i.e., men aged 65 years and over and women aged 60 years and over) while it has been estimated that this figure is likely to rise to 16½ per cent during the next 15 years.

This represents 8.6 million people in England and Wales. But the *largest increases are in the older age groups.* By 1986, there will be approximately 24 per cent more people aged 75 years and over. Yet the greatest increases are going to be seen in the very old age group—those aged 85 years and over. Now there are 1 in 104 persons in the country aged 85 years and over but *by 2001, this will be 1 in 65.*

There are many striking differences between the porportion of elderly men and women; 60 % of all old persons are women but this proportion is much greater in very old age (see Table 1, p. 20). Falling birth rates during this century have accentuated the rising proportion of old persons but the *biggest reason is associated with the increased life expectancy of young persons today.* The life expectancy of a boy today is 70 years and a girl 76. In 1911 the figures were 49 years and 52 years. Yet the life expectancy of a man aged 65 is now 12 years and a woman 16 years (compared with 11 and 12 years in 1911). There has always been much speculation about the *longevity of women compared with men.* There are probably many reasons—the majority of women have an active job looking after their home and also seem better able to withstand the effects of chronic crippling diseases which so often occur in old age.

Figure 16.1 shows clearly who the elderly lived with in 1976. These figures come from a survey of the elderly undertaken in England in 1976. Note that *94 per cent of all old persons live at home*; the remaining 6 per cent live in hostels, hospitals, etc., 28 per cent live alone and only 12 per cent are living with children. In fact two-thirds of all elderly households contain no one under the age of 65 years and one-third of the elderly have never had children or their children have not survived—they have no near immediate next generation family.

Disability among the elderly

The incidence of physical and mental disability among the elderly is high. About 65 per cent of all physically disabled persons are aged 65

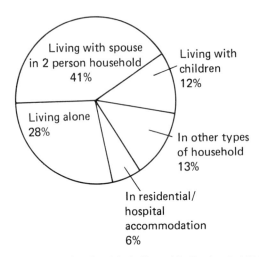

Fig. 16.1 Who the elderly live with, England, 1976

years and over. There is also a higher rate of mental illness in the elderly than in any other age group. The survey showed that 4 per cent of all persons aged 65 years and over were bedfast but *this figure rose to 20 % of those aged 85 years and over.* Of those who are not bedfast, 2 per cent have difficulty in seeing and 3 per cent in hearing. Reference has already been made to the fact that most blind persons are aged over 65 years of age. It will be clear that doctors and social workers meet many case problems in the elderly. Because so many old people live at home, *domiciliary services in both the medical and social fields are very important* if the likelihood of illness, accident or other problems is to be reduced.

Prevention of social and medical problems in old age

The avoidance of many problems in the elderly lies in various preventive steps including the earliest possible recognition of symptoms and social difficulties.

Advice to the elderly

Each local authority Social Services Department employs social workers and social work assistants who can help old people with advice and, if need be, visit them at home. This advisory work is carried out in very close association with many other persons working in the community and especially with those in the primary health care team—doctors, health visitors and home nurses. Links are also maintained with clergymen, voluntary workers, friendly visitors and community workers so that old people in need of special help can be found quickly. Any old person living alone (and in some towns and cities these represent 28 per cent of all old people) is always at special risk. Special alarms can be fixed (see page 248) but neighbours must play their part. Any person living near such an old person should in some way ensure daily that the old person is all right. In country villages and small towns, such surveillance is natural and tragedies rarely occur; however in large cities old people living alone are at much greater risk.

Planning for retirement

Many of the difficulties can be eased by some degree of *planning for old age*. Most serious mistakes are made by people about to retire. All too often they move to some unknown seaside resort for their retirement and are disappointed and find it difficult to settle down. It must always be remembered that the older the person, the more difficult it is to readjust. Human friendships are worth much more in old age than being in some attractive place.

Housing in retirement

Not enough regard is given to the type of house needed in old age. Whatever its type—flat, house or bungalow—it should always:

(a) be sited on level ground. So many of the traditional seaside towns, popular with retired persons, are too hilly
(b) have an entrance which can be directly approached by car—i.e., a car should be able to drive up to the front door
(c) have a downstairs room which is capable of being turned into a bedroom
(d) have a downstairs lavatory and washbasin (a downstairs bath is most helpful but often not possible, although a shower is often practicable)
(e) have an effective, simple and automatic system of heating

These five points are connected with the inevitable fact that certain physical limitations will eventually develop as the person gets older. The aim must always be *to help old persons to remain independent in their own home for as long as possible.*

It is always important that, if the old person is living in a house which is obviously too large and unwieldly, he leaves it for a smaller home *early* in retirement or *preferably* before. Old people never like the disturbance of moving and it becomes more difficult as they increase in age. So each should, if possible, be settled in the last home by the age of 60.

It is a help to ensure that in some way the house is heated automatically by oil, gas or electricity. Many old people feel the cold acutely and the constant stoking of coal fires is not without its hazards as regards falling. The inability of an elderly person to arrange proper heating of the accommodation will eventually lead to the dangerous condition of hypothermia.

It is most important that relatives do not take the old person permanently into their home unless this is clearly inevitable. Many kindly relatives are tempted to do this as they feel the old person is barely capable of continuing to look after himself or herself. But independence is very precious, especially to old people. Relatives such as children who precipitately take their elderly parents into their homes, may soon find it is a great mistake as the old person is not happy and begins to cause many difficulties. It is far better to arrange for the old person to stay temporarily with relatives—say for two to three weeks—and for them to retain their own home and independence.

Sheltered housing

This means a flatlet or flat for old people with a *resident warden in attendance* to ensure that help is readily available in an emergency. A bell or alarm is fitted to each flatlet. Old people living in such accommodation are usually fairly frail but can look after themselves. Occasionally a midday meal is provided for them in a luncheon club close by.

Sheltered housing is provided either by housing authorities or in accommodation built by housing trusts or voluntary bodies. The Social Services Committee usually pays a sum of £50–£150 per year per unit of sheltered accommodation to help pay the cost of the warden and other amenities (such as special alarms or telephones).

Supportive housing

Some local authorities are now introducing special units—supportive housing—where even more support can be given to the frail elderly person than in sheltered housing. In addition to a midday meal 2–3 hours of domestic help is provided daily, yet the old person retains his own 'front door' and identity to a greater extent than in any hostel.

Interests, hobbies, part-time work

Once the old person has settled in his home, he should always be encouraged to cultivate some hobby, pastime or interest. This process should preferably have been started before retirement. It does not matter what type of extra activity is tackled provided that it gives a real sense of purpose.

It is always helpful to encourage an old person to do some voluntary work, such as helping other people (elderly, handicapped or children). Occasionally it may be possible to undertake some form of part-time job.

For those who are in some way handicapped, perhaps because of physical limitations, it is important to encourage the continuation of their usual activities for as long as possible. Thus, a retired person should always be encouraged to look after the house even if he is unable to do all the work.

Financial help—pensions and allowances

Pensions and extra financial help are not provided directly by local authorities, but by the Department of Health and Social Security. However, many old people need help in claiming their pensions and other allowances (see Chapter 18) and the social worker should be ready at all times to explain and assist. It is most important that maximum use is made of pensions and allowances and it is never safe to assume that every old person fully understands his entitlement. Many of the elderly only imperfectly understand the range of pensions available and it is essential for each nurse to realize this and therefore discuss the matter with elderly patients in hospital. There are two special forms of financial help which are often overlooked—*rent rebates* and *rate rebates*.

Rent rebates. Under the Housing Finance Act, 1972, local authority tenants can obtain a rent rebate (reduction in rent) when their gross income is below a certain level. In the case of elderly pensioners, whose sole income is an old age pension, this usually means that considerably lower rents are paid.

Rate rebates. There is also a national scheme of special rate rebates (reduction in rates payable) which are available to elderly persons over 65 years of age with low incomes. There is a special scale which enables old people on low incomes to be excused a substantial part of their rates.

Any social services department of a local authority will gladly explain to and help any elderly person who may not understand his entitlement and assist in making a claim.

Heating

For any elderly person on supplementary benefit an extra heating allowance of £2.05 or £5.05 may be paid according to health, mobility and state of the accommodation.

Community services available to assist the elderly living in their own homes

Numerous special services are supplied by the social services department to assist the elderly living in their own homes. In all instances, the constant aim is to ensure the old person remains as independent as possible. In most cases, it is important to provide such services early enough so that they can prevent more serious difficulties from developing. Community services include:

(1) Home helps (see page 266)

The main value of home helps is to assist old people within their own homes. It is usual for the home help, who is often a married woman, to do the housework, essential shopping and get the old person a meal. The home help should always help with those tasks that are beyond the old person's capacity—cleaning windows and some of the heaviest tasks within the home.

Home help service can be full-time or part-time but, apart from emergencies, most of the home helps visit two or three times per week spending 2–4 hours with the old person at each visit. Some Social Services Committees provide a free service but the majority make a charge for this service based on a sliding scale; the elderly person with a good income would pay the full charge, but for any elderly person whose sole source of income is his old age pension, the service is usually free.

The provision of home helps is a most valuable service to the elderly and enables many who would otherwise be too frail, to stay within their own home. An important part of any home help's duties is to observe the old person at home in a sensible but inconspicuous way so that adequate warning can be given if the individual is becoming too frail to manage on his own.

Applications for home helps should be made to the Director of Social Services or Area Social Services Officer (see page 178).

(2) Good neighbour schemes

A number of local authorities have introduced 'good neighbour' schemes in which arrangements are made for someone living close by to call on an elderly person to help with many simple tasks—shopping, lighting the fire, simple cooking and light housework. Usually a small recompense of approximately £4–5 is paid to the good neighbour if she is helping regularly. Such services are usually given free to the old person, but are not provided by all local authorities.

(3) Home care programmes

Elderly persons living on their own are particularly susceptible to rapid deterioration when they are discharged home from hospital after an illness. Recently, *home care* programmes have been devised to support old people at such times. A typical scheme provides a home help and meals service for 20 per cent of elderly patients discharged from hospital (selected from those at special risk) for four weeks following discharge. At the end of the four weeks, any further help needed is given through the normal home help service.

(4) Meals service

There are two types of meals services which social services departments provide:

(a) *Meals-on-wheels* provide a hot two course meal delivered to the home of the old person, usually three or six times per week depending on the need. A small charge is made for this service, which is heavily subsidized.

(b) *Luncheon clubs* are for less frail old people who attend at some local hall or club from three to six times a week and there obtain a hot meal. These luncheon clubs are especially useful as the old person is encouraged to meet others, gets exercise walking to the club and not only gets the benefit of a good hot meal, but has the opportunity to make friends. A similar charge is usually made for the meal at the luncheon clubs as for meals-on-wheels.

(5) Day care centres

These have been described as 'hostels with beds' as they are intended to look after frail elderly persons requiring the kind of care and attention which is usually provided in hostels but who can sleep at home. Transport collects an old person from home and brings him to the centre to spend the day there and takes him home in the evening. Meals are provided as well as other services (laundry, hairdressing, etc.).

This type of care is of particular value where a frail old person is living with younger relatives who go out to work during the day. It is also useful for the elderly person living alone and can prevent much loneliness as well as ensuring that the old person can remain satisfactorily at home without having to be admitted permanently to a hostel. It is usual for each old person to come to a day care centre two or three times per week. A small charge is usually made.

(6) Clubs and day centres

There are many types of clubs and day centres run by social services departments and by voluntary bodies (especially Age Concern). These provide a centre which the old person can visit at any time for company, a light meal, tea or coffee and, in many instances, carry out some handicraft. Many social services departments subsidize such clubs. Attendance is usually free, but charges are made for meals, etc.

(7) Holidays and outings

Most local authorities through their social services departments arrange special holidays and outings for old people and this is also widely supplemented by the work of voluntary bodies. Holidays are especially important to help the elderly living alone and also for those living with younger relatives, for holidays enable each to have a break. In this way, a holiday can be of great value to both the old person and the family with whom he is living.

Some local authorities own seaside holiday homes, but many rely on making block bookings at seaside resorts in the off-peak season—early in summer or in autumn.

(8) Bus passes and concessionary fares

Facilities for unrestricted free travel on buses in off-peak times of the day (0930 to 1630 hours) can do much to maintain the independence of old people. Many local authorities have introduced special schemes in which elderly people can obtain such a free pass while other local authorities provide a certain number of tokens which can be exchanged for bus tickets. Schemes vary in different parts of the country and are now mainly available to those aged 60 (women) and 65 (men) in receipt of a pension.

(9) British rail senior citizens railcard

British rail has a scheme whereby anyone of pension age (60 and over for women and 65 and over for men) can buy a social rail card. It lasts a year from the date purchased. There are 2 types:

(a) with the £7 Railcard (1983) 'awayday' return tickets are half price
(b) with a £12 Railcard (1983), ordinary single and return tickets are half price and in continental countries, there are reduced fares.

Health services for the elderly

All the community medical services provided by the general practitioners are available to the elderly person at no extra cost *for there is no charge for any prescription for women aged 60 and over and for men aged 65 and over.* In recognition of the extra medical work involved in providing medical services for the elderly, there is a special increased per capita fee paid to general practitioners for all patients on their lists aged 65 years and older. Social workers and health visitors usually work in very close association with general practitioners whether they are based on health centres or not. In this way, it is hoped that the supporting social services (described above) which are provided by local authority social services departments will be increasingly used.

Geriatric hospitals and geriatric wards in general hospitals are widely available for investigation, treatment and rehabilitation of the elderly. The main differences between geriatric and ordinary acute hospitals are the special facilities the geriatric hospital has for:

(a) linking up with social services—this is because the social factors in the life of the old person often determine the seriousness of the illness and the outlook

(b) emphasizing the importance of **active rehabilitation** for all elderly people treated. This is because there is a real danger that the bed rest necessitated in the treatment of the elderly will tend to prevent their full recovery unless very active steps are taken to assist them to become fully active during convalescence.

Day hospitals

Day hospitals have recently been developed to help with the rehabilitation of elderly patients. They act as a sort of half-way stage between hospitals and home. Patients are brought there by transport and returned home in the evening. Old people may attend daily or on a specified number of days per week; physiotherapy and occupational therapy services are usually provided.

The main value of day hospitals is:

1   they allow the old person to be safely discharged home earlier—in this way they encourage independence;
2   they assist with the active rehabilitation of the patient;
3   they help to establish a better link between the geriatric unit and the community services for the elderly.

Community hospitals

In country districts *community hospitals* have helped develop a day hospital approach for some of their patients. It is valuable if health visitors and social workers arrange to visit the day hospital periodically and in this way improve the co-ordination between the two services.

These hospitals also provide short term 'respite' care for bedridden elderly persons being looked after at home to give the family a short break. They also are very useful for terminal cases and are staffed by the local general practitioners.

Home nursing

Home or community nurses are provided by every DHA to give nursing care for the patient treated at home. Approximately 44 per cent treated are elderly and the home nurse has a special responsibility for helping bedridden frail elderly people being looked after in their own homes. A special soiled laundry service has been developed in many areas to ensure a daily clean change of linen.

Chiropody

At present this is provided by District Health Authorities. In many instances the service is given at luncheon clubs, day care centres, clubs or any centre where old people congregate.

Foot defects can have a serious effect on the mobility of an old person (see page 259). Most people would benefit from this service, but the shortage of chiropodists makes it necessary for health authorities to provide this service only to those with obvious foot problems. There are two main ways of doing this service:

(a) special chiropody sessions are arranged in clinics and old people's clubs, where chiropody treatment is provided. Health authorities also carry out home treatment where this is essential. In most instances, however, it is much better to give chiropody treatment at a nearby centre for this encourages the elderly person to get out a little. However, initial treatment may have to be undertaken at home if the old person's feet are too painful to let him reach the clinic.

(b) chiropody treatment may be arranged at the private surgeries of chiropodists. In this case, the health authority meets the total cost.

To obtain the maximum value, it is important that chiropody treatment is regularly arranged *once every six to eight weeks*, otherwise the condition of the old person's feet may very quickly deteriorate again. As many elderly people are living on small pensions and find it difficult to meet extra expenses, it is best if chiropody treatment for the aged is provided free of charge.

Special problems seen in the elderly living at home

Often an illness or accident is the starting point of rapid deterioration in any old person living at home. Because of this factor, *any illness in an old person* must be treated seriously even if it is trivial. Special steps must be taken to ensure that the old person is completely treated and rehabilitated.

Rehabilitation can be hastened by arranging for the old person, while recovering, to attend a rehabilitation unit run by a local authority or by a hospital. Physiotherapy and occupational therapy are most valuable to old people whose rheumatism or arthritis has inevitably been aggravated by staying in bed during an illness. Both physiotherapy and occupational therapy will help the old person to get moving again during convalescence.

Convalescence on return home can be aided by arranging a full-time home help for a fortnight, and then reducing the help, as the old person takes over the routine tasks. In this way, it is often possible to nurse an old person through a serious illness without eventual loss of function and independence.

Prevention of mental deterioration

The mental state of the vast majority of elderly people living at home is good. A recent survey showed that 82 per cent of the elderly at home were fully normal, with about 11 per cent showing minor problems, 4 per cent showing clear indication of mental breakdown and the remaining 3 per cent were classified as eccentrics.

There seems little doubt that an important factor in maintaining the *mental vigour of any old person* at home, is connected with living in the surroundings they have always been used to and of *having something useful to do*.

The memory of most elderly people is good except for minor difficulties of remembering names. When mental impairment occurs, memory is one of the first factors to be affected.

Domestic anxieties, loneliness and physical defects resulting in limitation of movement seem to induce mental failure. Anxieties in old age often are due to the old person not properly understanding certain financial or legal problems. Careful, patient explanation *by the health visitor or social worker* and the sorting out of pension and legal difficulties (rent, lease or will) can often do much to help. Some old people may worry excessively about financial problems and may increasingly stint themselves trying to save, when their financial circumstances are quite sound. This excessive anxiety about money often tends to get worse as age increases and is best prevented by ensuring that the old person fully understands how many of the financial worries are groundless. It is important to point out that today the same type of provision is made in all old people's homes whether the full cost is paid or whether the old person is living on a pension. *Much tact and patience are needed, however,* and it must always be remembered that the old people today, are a generation brought up before the concept of social security, and there is often a deep seated fear of 'living on charity'.

There seems to be a close association between the development of emotional disturbance in old people and either the death of a husband, or wife, or a severe fall. After either event, therefore, considerable help will be needed to assist the old person to overcome the effects.

When mental deterioration in the elderly living at home occurs, the symptoms often include:

1　*Change in outlook of the old person*—either towards apathy or agitation.
2　*Eating habits may change*—and often the old person becomes very fussy and will eat very little.
3　*Depression* is commoner—as well as occasional outbreaks of verbal aggression making the old person much more difficult to live with.
4　*Memory*—there is an early failure of memory noted.
5　*Talk*—any tendency to talk a lot, a characteristic of many old people, soon disappears.
6　Worries which may become morbidly increased.
7　There is a marked loss in the ability of the old person to look after himself.

It is always valuable to recognize promptly impending early mental deterioration in the elderly at home, as it makes early treatment possible and may prevent, in this way, a serious and perhaps final mental breakdown.

Loneliness in the elderly

One of the most pathetic complications of old age is loneliness. It is not always connected with living alone, rather the very lonely old person seems to have cut himself or herself off from the world.

Many social and health factors are usually connected with the problem. The most serious is the sudden loss of a beloved husband or wife. Men seem to suffer from extreme loneliness more than women. Extreme loneliness in widowers occurs even when they are not living alone—in other words, loneliness does not seem to result directly from their social circumstances.

Loneliness of some degree probably occurs in about 20 per cent of elderly persons. There are many causes—bereavement, departure of children, absence of hobbies, limitation of physical activity.

It is never easy to prevent loneliness developing. Increasing social contact may occasionally help. Another approach is in some way to encourage the old person to understand that he is of some value to others and especially to younger people. Loneliness is so often 'an attitude of mind' in which the old person loses interest and becomes isolated.

Although not invariable, any old person who has varying interests and hobbies is less likely to suffer from extreme loneliness even if their circumstances may suddenly change. Thus the encouragement of widespread hobbies and interests among young and middle-aged persons will do much to prevent extreme loneliness later in old age.

Home accidents

Old people living at home, either with a family or on their own, are *more liable to have accidents*—particularly to falls. Recent surveys have shown that about 35 per cent of elderly people are liable to fall. In any elderly person, a fall is likely to be more serious than a similar accident in a younger person, both because (a) it is more likely to result in serious injury, especially in the development of various fractures, and (b) it may also precipitate senile decay.

Women are more liable to falls than men and the tendency to fall increases with age. Sheldon in his classic survey in Wolverhampton classified home falls in old people in four ways:

1 **Falls associated with attacks of vertigo**. A sudden attack of vertigo, dizziness, occurs in the course of movement and unless there is a solid object immediately at hand, the old person falls headlong.
2 **Falls associated with an increased liability to trip**. Women seem particularly liable to trip over small objects. Many old people who, when younger never had a tendency to trip, find as they grow old, they are much more likely to do so. They trip more easily over small objects or if there is a trivial unevenness in the floor level.
3 **Falls due to difficulty in recovering balance**. There seems no doubt that many old people find their power in recovering their balance after trivial false movement is much impaired compared with their ability to do so when younger.
4 **Falls due to sudden collapse, or to legs giving way**. This seems particularly to occur in very old people over the age of 80. The old

person suddenly collapses and often is unable to move for some time afterwards even if he or she has not been injured in the fall.

Many of these falls can be prevented and their effect diminished. The possibility—and in old people over 85 probability—of a fall should always be considered by those looking after the old person.

The following steps should be taken to diminish the chance of falls:

(a) An old person increasingly depends on *sight* to maintain balance, as his labyrinthine function is often faulty. Thus, an old person who may be quite steady in daylight may be very liable to fall in the dark. This should be explained to the old person who should always ensure that there is adequate light throughout his home. It is particularly important to see that the lighting of passages or staircases is really good—at least a 60 watt bulb should be used.

(b) The likelihood of a tendency to increased tripping should always be remembered and care must be taken to ensure that floor fittings, carpets, linoleum, rugs, etc., are securely fastened. In families where old people live, children must not leave toys around on floors over which the old person is likely to walk. There should never be loose electric flex across a floor.

(c) Wherever possible, an old person should learn to walk with some support from a solid object—banister, handrail, chair, table, furniture, especially if it is known that there is a liability to fall or should constantly use a walking aid such as a Zimmer.

Intelligent anticipation of the causes of a fall can do much to prevent one—the result of which could easily mean the death of the elderly person.

Rheumatism and arthritis

Many elderly people have some degree of *rheumatism* or *degenerative arthritis*. It is difficult to ascertain the exact amount of these conditions, as the criteria of diagnosis varies with different observers. Surveys have reported that 50 per cent to 80 per cent of elderly people living at home complain of rheumatic symptoms of one kind and another.

It is interesting that many elderly persons, even with marked osteoarthritis, find that however painful initial movement may be, the more active they are around the house the less problem the arthritis is. For this reason, enforced activity in an elderly woman still looking after her home, often prevents her condition from deteriorating. With this in mind, all forms of activity—physiotherapy, the carrying out of some simple occupation, occupational therapy, are all useful in preventing further limitation.

The success of *hip replacement surgery* has been very marked and any elderly person who is seriously crippled with degenerative joint disease of the hips should always consider a hip replacement operation. In most cases such an operation will render them completely mobile for 10–15 years.

Some of the worst cases of degenerative arthritis occur in fat people. The prevention of obesity in younger people will reduce the likelihood of a severe arthritis developing at a later age.

In all instances where there is a limitation in the range of movement of an old person, the various social services designed to help with their feeding problems should be used—such as meals-on-wheels; with housework problems—home helps; and with shopping difficulties—friendly visitors; are most important in avoiding the development of other medical problems.

Foot defects

Foot defects very often cause serious problems in old people. The types of abnormalities include ingrowing toe-nails, flat foot, hallux valgus, bunions and corns, and hammer toes.

At least half of the old people living at home suffer from some form of foot defect. In many of them, this leads to pain on walking and consequently usually produces some limitation of movement. This can be of a serious degree and may result occasionally in the old person becoming more or less house bound.

Most of the foot conditions found in old people can be prevented at least from causing serious effects by arranging radical treatment for the more disabling conditions, and for the minor conditions, regular chiropody (see page 254) and by teaching foot hygiene.

Hypothermia

This is a serious condition in which the body cannot maintain correct temperature control and consequently loses heat, especially in winter time. It is very important that the methods used in diagnosing this condition are fully understood by all people looking after the elderly. Hypothermia is a dangerous condition if not recognized early and is particularly likely to occur in old people living alone in houses that are inadequately heated.

Hypothermia is NOT only seen in old people living in cold homes (although such conditions will always make it more likely). It may suddenly and dangerously occur in an elderly person who has been taken ill suddenly (as in pneumonia), even though he is seated in a chair in a room which is not unduly cold. It can also occur after strokes, or after a heart attack in which the old person may sit quietly in a chair for hours on end.

Whatever the cause, it is *most important* that the condition is *recognized early* and that all staff dealing with the elderly know the early signs of hypothermia. The old person *does not usually look cold* and certainly does not shiver. The hands and face often look warm and are red or reddish purple in colour. The individual is often drowsy and very inactive and speech may become slow and slurred. The hands, feet and face feel cold and the body temperature (as measured on a specially low recording thermometer) is usually well below 35°C (95°F).

Once the condition is recognized, emergency treatment must be started; treatment is often difficult and unsatisfactory. Rapid warming is *very dangerous to old people with hypothermia* and therefore must be avoided at all costs. The aim should be to limit the warming up of the old person to approximately 0.6°C (1°F) per hour. The room temperature should be kept warm and a few extra blankets should be applied but no direct heat.

Prevention of hypothermia. The prevention of hypothermia involves more than anything else realizing that the condition can develop insidiously. All those looking after old people therefore should be on their guard. In particular three important factors should be stressed;

1 ensuring that old people are accommodated in warm conditions;
2 encouraging elderly people to move around and not allowing them to sit all day even if they are in a relatively warm room;
3 always realizing that hypothermia is very likely to occur in any illness in an old person. For this reason anyone nursing an old person, especially in their own home, should always be on the look-out.

Cardiovascular disease

About 18 per cent of elderly people are limited in their activity on account of cardiovascular disease. Just under 5 per cent are limited to the house, while 13 per cent found some limitation in their activity out of doors. *Angina of effort* is the commonest single factor, with *pulmonary heart failure* and *cerebrovascular accidents* being other reasons for limitation. Angina may be helped by modern heart surgery in which a coronary artery transplant is carried out—this may be specially useful in the younger elderly person with angina of effort.

A great deal can also be done to minimize the effect of many of these conditions by improving social conditions. The position of the home of an elderly person often has a marked effect upon the amount of limitation caused to anyone with even an early stage of heart failure and its effects. Any hill which has to be negotiated is likely to have a most limiting effect on the heart patient. Stairs in the house too are most undesirable. The best home for any aged person is on the flat, with direct access to the front door by car so that an elderly patient with heart disease can move from his house without having to go up an incline. A bungalow is much better than a house as it has no stairs.

Hearing loss and vertigo

About 30 per cent of the elderly at home have some degree of hearing loss, but there is a much higher incidence of deafness in the oldest age group—in those aged 80 and over the incidence of deafness approaches 60 per cent.

In many cases it is impossible to prevent the deafness itself, but a great deal can be done to prevent its worst effects by the provision and maintenance of a hearing aid. Many old people who are deaf have developed deafness over many years and have got used to a number of its great disadvantages.

However, *deafness* more than any other single cause, *leads to isolation of the old person*—isolation from the easy and natural social contact of chatting to people. For the family living with a deaf old person, who can hear very little, the difficulty of communication greatly adds to the problems created by the elderly person. Mutual resentment soon follows with a general deterioration in the relationship between the family and the old person.

A properly fitted and maintained hearing aid may prevent such a situation developing and, in this way, avoid much unnecessary unhappiness to the old person. Patience and encouragement are needed, otherwise the patient soon gets fed up with the minor difficulties of the aid and ceases to use it.

Vertigo, dizziness, can be an important and distressing symptom seen in some old people. It is most likely to occur in women aged 85 and over but, although found in men up to 79, is rarely seen in men over 80 years of age. In the extreme cases, there is little done to prevent its occurrence except to ensure that no old person, who is very liable to such attacks, lives alone. The extreme likelihood of falls makes great care necessary. In the less severe cases, a full investigation should always be carried out, as well as arranging for all the precautions already mentioned to prevent falls. In particular, it must always be remembered that old people with vertigo are likely to have *great difficulty in the dark*. It is, therefore, most important that they never get up from bed at night without turning on the light which should be a bright one. To ensure that the old person can easily find the switch on awaking, it is wise to have some form of night light in the bedroom.

Visual defects

It is usual for most old people to have to rely on spectacles to overcome visual defects. Well over 90 per cent of elderly men and women require spectacles for near vision and between 50 per cent and 60 per cent for distant vision.

Recent surveys have shown a different assessment regarding the incidence of unsatisfactory spectacles. It is, however, still clear that a considerable proportion of elderly people are not obtaining the help they should from their spectacles because they are unsuitable and need changing.

Ignorance may still play a part, for some old people may not know how important it is to *retest the sight of any person regularly*. To avoid this problem, those visiting old poeple should try to ensure that their vision is tested every two to three years. It may not be enough just to advise retesting, it may be necessary for a social worker or health visitor to arrange an appointment and to take the old person by car to the optician.

Blindness or near blindness only occurs in 1 to 2 per cent of the elderly living at home. The individual problems of blindness have been discussed in detail in Chapter 14 (pages 214–219).

Nutrition of the aged

Health is only possible provided there is an adequate and well-balanced diet. This is true of all ages but the maintenance of an adequate nutrition is particularly important in all elderly persons.

A recent survey showed that, in the opinion of the investigators, 17 per cent of elderly men and 22 per cent of elderly women had a poor level of nutrition. Foods requiring some preparation are eaten less by old people living alone than when they are living in families or as a married couple.

Cases of extremely poor nutrition in old people are usually connected with an *elderly person living alone* who has lost interest in preparing meals, or who is not having any outside meals. Occasionally extreme difficulty of mobility (from any cause) may lead to inadequate shopping. With the very busy streets of many towns, old people may find it increasingly difficult to cross the road and if an essential food shop—say a greengrocer—is on the other side of the road, then the old person may unnecessarily restrict her diet just because shopping is such an ordeal. The realization that such a simple cause may start a chain of events, which could eventually lead to a severe state of malnutrition, should be sufficient to suggest a simple remedy—an arrangement with a friendly neighbour to help with the shopping.

All those who are, in any way, working with old people whether as doctors, home nurses, health visitors, social workers, voluntary workers or even just neighbours and friends, should always remember that, particularly in the case of an old person living alone, the monotony of preparing meals for oneself can soon lead to inadequate and quite unbalanced diet.

The remedy is to try and make immediate arrangements:

1 for the old person to go, if able, to an old persons club for three or four
   good meals per week; (see page 252) or
2 to arrange for *meals-on-wheels* service to be delivered three or more
   times a week; (see page 251) or
3 to arrange a part-time home help service for the elderly person. Part of
   the duties of the home help would be to cook a hot meal for the old
   person when she visited him (see page 266).

Pulmonary disease in the elderly

Bronchitis and *emphysema* together with bronchial spasm are the chief
causes of respiratory illness in the elderly.

About 40 per cent of elderly people have some degree of bronchitis with
chronic cough; these figures are from industrial areas and are likely to be
lower for rural ones. Men suffer more from this than women. About *4 per
cent of the elderly are severely disabled by bronchitis.*

The prevention of bronchitis in the elderly is, of course, the same as
prevention of the disease in adults. The bronchitis of the aged is only a
later stage of the bronchitis in the middle aged.

Apart from the particular hazards of dust in certain occupations
already discussed, there is no doubt that *persistent cigarette smoking* is the
main cause of much of the irritation, chronic cough and expectoration. It
cannot be too strongly stressed that any adult who is a smoker with a
chronic cough and with winter attacks of bronchitis, *must give up smoking
at once to prevent slowly deteriorating and progressive chronic bronchitis
developing*, with all its crippling invalidism. Thus, the prevention of the
problem of bronchitis in old age often rests with stopping smoking as an
adult. If an old person stops smoking, it usually helps but if he has already
developed a severe degree of chronic bronchitis, it may be impossible to
halt the disease.

Prolapse and stress incontinence

About 12 to 15 per cent of married women over the age of 60 years
probably suffer from some degree of prolapse with stress incontinence of
urine. The highest incidence is seen in women who have had many
pregnancies. Immediate gynaecological investigation should always be
carried out as, in many, a simple operation can help.

Enlarged prostate

About 25 per cent of men over the age of 65 years have symptoms of
enlarged prostate. Symptoms in these cases usually include:

(a) frequency of micturition by day or night
(b) dribbling with overflow
(c) urinary incontinence both occasional and regular.

The prevention of both conditions consists of *early diagnosis and treatment*. It must be remembered that symptoms of prostatic enlargement can often be greatly helped by hormone therapy.

There is nothing worse than incontinence and it is also important to realize that radical operative treatment is nearly always worth while even with the very elderly, for the results are often excellent.

Incontinence is a difficult problem with some elderly people. Its management involves:

(a) making certain that medical or surgical treatment will not help;

(b) encouraging the old person to empty their bladder regularly. There is much evidence that a number of those who suffer from incontinence just 'forget' to go regularly to the lavatory. Therefore in hostels where attendants remind the old people from time to time the level of incontinence is always less;

(c) the use of suitable clothing. A number of old people have, urgency and cannot undo their clothing in time. There is a wide range of special clothing designed and available from the Disabled Living Foundation or aids centres which can help in this problem. Buttons are replaced by 'velcro' and many garments have special front openings although they are designed in such a way as to look normal.

Residential services

Hostels for old people

Every local authority has to provide through its Social Services Committee hostels for elderly persons. Most of the modern hostels are specially designed and newly built. A few have been converted from large houses.

The modern old person's hostel is usually designed for from 35 to 55 old people. Hostels larger than this are not popular as it would be difficult to maintain a friendly personal atmosphere in them. Each new hostel has a majority of single rooms but a few twin-bedded ones. A hostel usually has lounges of varying size, situated on each floor. A lift must be provided so that all the accommodation is of the 'ground floor type', in other words, can be reached without the old person having to climb any stairs.

A resident matron and staff are in charge, and minor illnesses are usually looked after by them, but in the case of more prolonged or serious illness, the old person should be admitted to hospital and when fit again, return to the hostel.

Each hostel provides a high standard of care for those living there and it is usual for all the needs of the old people to be provided, including clothing.

One very special arrangement in old persons' hostels is that every old person contributes to their cost. Each hostel has a standard charge—a usual present day (1983) figure is approximately £100 per week which represents the economic cost of keeping an old person in the hostel. Each old person is asked if they can afford to pay this charge. If they can, they do. If not, then each old person must pay a proportion of their old age pension or Social Security allowance. The statutory minimum charge is £26.30 (1983) per week. This portion is calculated so that the old person is always left with £6.55 (1983) a week pocket money for personal spending. The local authority is responsible for the additional cost.

Old people's homes today should be happy places. They, of necessity, take the frailer old people who cannot manage at home.

Hostels are also provided by many voluntary and church organizations. In many instances, local authorities will assist the voluntary body by paying a per-capita grant based on the weekly cost of keeping the elderly person.

Emergency compulsory removal of an old person from home

Occasionally it is necessary to consider removing compulsorily an old person from home because it is dangerous for him to stay at home and he refuses to enter a hospital or old person's hostel. Fortunately few elderly persons are removed in this way as most readily agree or can be persuaded. Cases that have to be moved are those who have badly neglected themselves and include those suffering from late cancers and others who are afraid to go into hospital.

Action is taken under s. 47 of the National Assistance Act, 1948 and the Amendment Act, 1951, which gives power for the compulsory removal of aged and certain other people to hospitals or other institutions. It is only possible to remove those who are:

(i) suffering from grave chronic disease or being aged, infirm or physically incapacitated, are living in insanitary conditions; *and*

(ii) are unable to devote to themselves, and are not receiving from other persons, proper care and attention.'

The Social Services Department arranges the removal but first the District Medical Officer must arrange for a doctor to certify that it is in the interests of the person to do this. If the magistrate (or Court) is satisfied, the removal to hospital or hostel is then carried out.

17
Other Community Social Services

Home helps

Every Social Services authority (County Councils, Metropolitan District Councils and London Boroughs) has a duty to provide a home help service adequate for the needs of the area (s. 13 of the Health Services and Public Health Act, 1968).

The object of the home help service is to provide assistance in the home where because of age, acute or chronic illness (physical or mental), the housewife cannot look after the home. The service is also used in some maternity cases.

The majority of the work of the home help services is with the care of *elderly people* (see page 250) but other groups are also covered including *chronic illness*, and the younger physically handicapped. Home helps also assist families with young children especially when sudden illness arises, or when either parent is away, perhaps in hospital, and when such help would enable the parent to rejoin the family more quickly.

In looking after some handicapped children, home help care is most useful for it can allow a mother more time to spend teaching her child. This is especially important for a child who is born deaf, for a home help provided while the child is aged $1\frac{1}{2}$ to 5 years can be of great assistance by allowing the mother to spend much more time teaching the child lip reading. While the mother spends say 4–5 hours solely with the child, the home help is assisting with housework and shopping.

About 88 per cent of the work carried out by home helps is with the elderly: nearly 6 per cent with chronic sick cases and the remainder for other reasons including a few maternity cases and the mentally handicapped. Approximately 665 000 persons receive home help assistance each year in England.

It is usual to make a charge for the service, but there is a sliding scale according to income; those on social security or those receiving the old age pension as their only income are given the service free.

Most of the 92 000 home helps at present working in England do so part-time. The duties of a home help vary with each case, but include many of the normal tasks carried out by the housewife—cleaning rooms, preparing food and meals, shopping, lighting fires and, in a family, looking after the children. A few social service authorities provide free home helps for all clients.

Home help service can be provided full-time or part-time to the client depending on the circumstances. Apart from emergency work, most of the service by home helps is usually provided part-time, perhaps amounting to two or three sessions per week. This is particularly important when an elderly person is helped in this way over a long period for it is *essential to encourage the old person to continue to do as much housework as possible herself*, and, in this way, keep active as long as possible.

In emergency illness or maternity cases, a full-time help for a short period may enable a young family to be kept together and thus avoid the need to take children into short-term care. This type of support is particularly valuable where there are no relatives or family to help (apart from the father of the family who has to continue to go to work).

Links between home helps and a co-ordinated domiciliary team

The home help soon gets to know the client or family she is visiting very well and learns a great deal about their personal problems. It is, therefore, important that *all home helps form part of a balanced and co-ordinated domiciliary social work team* and, in particular, *work in close contact with social workers*.

Because of this, most social services departments have arranged for home help services to be organized within their area social services teams. In this way, any useful information the home help has learnt about her charges can easily be passed on to the social workers so that the fullest possible social support can be arranged.

For the same reasons, the local organizer of home helps must *co-ordinate closely with general practitioners, home nurses* and many others who need the assistance of home helps from time to time in their practices.

Occasionally the home help has to tackle a particularly difficult, dirty or heavy task to clean up a home which has become extremely dirty due to the neglect or illness of the occupant. Many social services departments arrange special teams to do this special work and many provide special equipment. It is usual for those tackling such exceptionally difficult tasks to be given extra remuneration for such work.

'Good neighbour schemes'

Usually the demand for home helps outstrips the provision and some authorities have experimented with alternative methods of help such as 'good neighbour schemes'. In this local volunteers are sought, often from among fit older people, who will agree to carry out a number of light duties—shopping, cooking, light cleaning, etc. Most schemes rely on recruiting such volunteers from members of the public living close by so that no travelling is involved.

Most schemes arrange for the volunteer to be paid a small sum, say £4–5 per week as an honorarium, provided help is given on most or all days of the week.

Care of homeless families

Since the introduction of the Housing (Homeless Persons) Act, 1977, the main responsibility and duty for providing temporary or permanent accommodation for those who are homeless rests with the local housing authority (metropolitan and other district councils). Social Services authorities are required to co-operate by giving homeless clients support and advice.

The 1977 Act introduced 2 new concepts:

(a) those who are homeless are divided into *priority cases* and others. Priority cases indicate anyone who has one or more children living with them, anyone made homeless because of an emergency (fire, flood etc.), and any household which includes one or more people who are elderly or mentally handicapped or suffer from a physical disability. Battered wives and pregnant women are also priority cases.

(b) the homeless are divided into those made homeless by chance and those made homeless intentionally.

Duties of housing authorities to those who are homeless

A. For those with a priority need. Provided the homelessness is not intentional, the housing authority has a duty to provide permanent accommodation which enables the family to live together as soon as possible.

If the homelessness is intentional, the local housing authority is obliged:

1   to provide accommodation for the household on a temporary basis;
2   to provide advice and assistance.

B. For those who do not have a priority need (whether intentional or not). For those cases, the housing authority have a responsibility to give advice and assistance as they consider appropriate in any attempts the homeless person may make to obtain or retain accommodation for himself. The Code of Guidance published with the Act indicates that such assistance should include registering the family on the housing list, giving assistance through a housing aid centre or referring the case to housing associations or voluntary bodies. Advice should also be given regarding lists of accommodation agencies, hostels and possible accommodation in the privately owned sector.

Many homeless families need much continuous help and support. Some are difficult to help—perhaps due to the low intelligence of the mother or father. Careful after care work often needs to be carried out after rehousing, otherwise the family may inevitably fall into debt and repeat their mistakes.

Initially some homeless families are rehoused in sub-standard housing and then progress towards normal council housing. This usually occurs once the family has shown themselves capable of managing their own affairs. Even at this stage, such families need much support from social workers, family service units, health visitors and others.

Prevention of homelessness

The prevention of homelessness is in many ways more important than its treatment. There are two special problems, (1) the avoidance of large rent arrears, and (2) the support and help given to homeless families immediately after their rehousing. The avoidance of large rent arrears involves a number of actions which should be taken by housing and social services departments without having to resort to eviction. The following are important:

1 An early warning system after a few missed payments should be instituted to enable special arrangements for rent collection to be made, and for social services advice to be sought.
2 If rent arrears are still accumulating, housing authorities should check whether the tenants are eligible for rent and rate rebates.
3 There should be a vigorous pursuit of rent arrears and this should include selective visiting in certain areas to prevent the arrears becoming greater.
4 If the family are receiving supplementary benefit, then this will contain a sum equivalent to the rent and arrangements can be made in suitable cases for this to be paid directly to the local authority.
5 If there are serious family and social problems, it may be possible to assist by payment of rent arrears, using powers of s. 1 of the Children's and Young Persons Act 1963.

Transfer to cheaper accommodation to help reduce the rent problems. Care has to be taken in such cases to see that there is not undue concentration of families in social difficulties.

Family planning (see pages 50–1) in all homeless families should always be carefully considered as too many children at too short intervals in any family are likely to aggravate problems. In the most intractable problem families, it is best to arrange a domiciliary family planning service to ensure the mother receives correct family planning advice, otherwise few will attend clinics (see page 51).

Bed and breakfast accommodation. In some urban areas, there is a grave shortage of temporary accommodation and families have to be housed for the time being in 'bed and breakfast' accommodation. This arrangement *must* be made by the Social Services Department (under the Children and Young Persons Act, 1963). It is always an unsatisfactory expedient and housing authorities should always attempt to rehouse such families as quickly as possible. Generally, since the Act, bed and breakfast has been considerably reduced.

Care of unsupported mothers

The care of the unsupported mother (including the unmarried mother) is also the responsibility of social services departments who can make arrangements, often in conjunction with voluntary bodies, for the residential care of some mothers. As with other types of homelessness, it is important to do everything to educate the mother to prevent further problems. It follows from this that *the unmarried mother needs a considerable amount of supporting social work*; most will also require much advice and teaching which is best arranged by social workers in conjunction with the health visitors (see page 48).

Hospital social workers

In the reorganization of 1974, the control of hospital social workers was transferred from the health services to local authority Social Services Departments. The number of hospital social workers has steadily increased in the last 25 years and their tasks have altered. At present there are approximately 2200 hospital social workers and most of these work in district general hospitals or in geriatric and paediatric units. Those who work in psychiatric hospitals are usually specially qualified *psychiatric social workers.*

There are four main areas of work for hospital social workers:

(1) **Medical casework** concerned with the adjustment of the patient and his family to the patient's disease. This is the largest and most important aspect of hospital social work. It mainly involves working with the patient in hospital (including in-patient and out-patient work) but may also necessitate the hospital social worker visiting the patient's home. All types of cases are covered, work with children including non-accidental injury cases; much work is also undertaken with the elderly, many of whom live alone and are consequently very vulnerable (see page 255). Terminal cases are included, especially carcinoma. Illness in the parent of a one-parent family often produces many extra difficulties which the hospital social worker will try to solve. Another important group of cases are accident patients and especially those suffering from chronic disabling diseases including rheumatoid arthritis. Many social problems occur in mental illness and the role of the hospital social worker in such cases is often a crucial one.

(2) **Environmental help**—arranging how the patient's home can be improved to help him cope with the illness. This may involve the complete rehousing of the patient or the adaptation of the home either structurally or by the introduction of certain aids.

(3) Arrangements for **immediate assistance to the patient or his/her relatives**. This includes financial help, convalescent arrangements, provision of escorts or accommodation for relatives visiting dangerously-ill relatives.

(4) **Liaison** with various other social work agencies (including the Social Services Department of the area where the patient lives) to enable long-term care and rehabilitation of the patient.

Alcoholism

Alcoholism can be defined as dependence upon alcohol to such a degree that the person shows noticeable mental disturbance or an interference with bodily or mental health. Alcoholism is both a medical and social problem in its origins and manifestations—it interferes with interpersonal relations and with the normal economic and social functioning of the alcoholic and his family.

It is estimated that there are about 350 000 to 400 000 alcoholics in England and Wales. Recently there has been evidence that the incidence is increasing especially in women and young persons.

Causes of alcoholism

There are many causes of alcoholism. Social factors are very important and there is a higher incidence in people who are single, widowed or divorced. The average age for men who become alcoholics is the mid-forties while in women it is higher. Certain occupations are at high risk—commercial travellers, business executives, publicans, seamen and doctors. No particular personality is specially susceptible although a higher incidence occurs in both excessively shy people and gregarious extraverts.

Types of alcoholism

There are 2 main types:

1   *Alcohol addiction*—persons who cannot go for long without a drink of alcohol or who get withdrawal symptoms if they stop drinking.
2   *Chronic alcoholism* in which serious physical and mental symptoms are important features. Loss of appetite and poor food intake encourage the development of cirrhosis of the liver and peripheral

neuropathy. Severe memory loss is often present and dementia may occur. Withdrawal symptoms may also occur (including delirium tremens).

Treatment, rehabilitation and after-care

Early diagnosis is always very important. Increasing absenteeism, decline in job efficiency, increasing marital disharmony and self-neglect are always very suggestive. Memory loss, misinterpretations and feelings of guilt and low self-esteem should raise suspicions. Ill-effects in other members of the family, especially wives, may occur.

Treatment is aimed at reversing the damage to the physical, mental and social life of the alcoholic and *then* to deal with the underlying addiction. Eighteen special alcoholism units (including detoxification centres) have been set up and many mental hospitals also provide treatment.

Once successful treatment has ended, relapses are common unless a careful rehabilitation process is started. Doctors should work closely with social workers from either the Social Services Department or voluntary bodies in the follow-up. Special *hostels* or *day centres* may have to be used. As many alcoholics have lost their job the Disablement Resettlement Officer should be able to assist.

Many voluntary bodies such as various Councils for Alcoholism and Alcoholics Anonymous, can give useful support.

18
Social Security

A very wide range of Social Security benefits are available and most patients that the nurse deals with in her practice will be entitled to one of these benefits. Social Security has become very complicated and to make things even more difficult for the student, most governments are constantly changing the range and amount of allowance payable. It is, therefore, *important that every nurse understands the basic* allowances or benefits which are available, and also *consults the excellent booklet published by the Department of Health and Social Security* currently called 'Which benefit?' and obtainable free from local Social Security offices to check the latest details.

In this chapter, an attempt is made to introduce the nurse to the *range of* Social Security benefits available. The list given is not intended to be a complete one, but does cover the most important aspects of social security. It was up to date at the time of writing.

Benefits fall into three main types:

1 **Non-contributory**
   These are available to everyone who qualifies and do not depend on the individual having contributed for a set time into the social security system.
2 **Contributory**
   To qualify for these, two factors must be satisfied:
   (i) that the individual has contributed a minimum number of weekly contributions over a set period of time, and
   (ii) that his circumstances satisfy the requirements for each particular benefit.
3 Provided the individual qualifies, **an entitlement to certain services** at no cost or at reduced cost.

Non-contributory benefits

There are twelve main non-contributory benefits:

(a) Child Benefit
(b) Family Income Supplement
(c) Supplementary Benefits
(d) Attendance Allowance
(e) Mobility Allowance
(f) Non-contributory invalidity pension

(g) Pensions for persons over 80 years of age
(h) Guardian's allowance
(i) Various industrial injury benefits including injury benefit, disablement benefit, industrial death benefit
(j) Invalid care allowance
(k) Employment rehabilitation allowance
(l) Criminal injuries compensation.

(a) Child Benefit

Since 1977, a new social security benefit called child benefit has replaced family allowances. It is payable to *all* children including the first or only child. The children must be under school leaving age (16 years) or under the age of 19 and at school, college or university full-time. If the child is receiving non-contributory invalidity pension, he/she cannot also receive child benefit.

The claim for child benefit must be made by a person responsible for the child. Usually this will be the mother of the child (whether married or not). If the child lives with people who are not the parents but who share the responsibility, they can decide for themselves who should claim or ask the local Social Security Office. Child Benefit is tax free. The rates of child benefit in 1985 are £6.85 for each child.

Extra benefit for children (£7.65 in 1985) can be claimed by those looking after children and who are also claiming invalidity benefits, retirement and widow's pensions and invalidity care allowance.

One parent benefit of £4.25 (1985) can be claimed on top of child benefit for the first child of a lone parent who is bringing up the child but who is NOT receiving widow's benefits.

Child benefit is NOT payable for any week in which a child is in the care of a local authority or to a foster parent in receipt of a boarding out allowance. If a child returns home (for a holiday or on trial) child benefit will be payable for any completed week.

(b) Family income supplement (FIS)

This is a benefit to assist families whose normal gross weekly income is very low. Anyone, including a single person, with at least one dependent child can claim *provided he or she is in full-time work* or, for a couple, the man is in full-time work (this means 30 or more hours per week). All children who are normally living with the claimant can be included if under 16 years or aged 16 and over if still at school.

The rate of supplement equals one half of the difference between the family's normal gross income and the prescribed amount decided by Parliament. In 1983, this prescribed amount was £85.50 for a family with one child plus £9.50 for each additional child. Family allowances and other sources of income—such as wife's earnings—are included in the total income but *the income of any child is not.* The maximum supplement (1983) is £22.00 per week for families with one child increasing by £2.00 for each additional child.

Family Income Supplement can be claimed on forms obtainable from local Social Security Offices or Post Offices. Details of the last five weeks' income will be needed. *Note*: Any person awarded family income supplement is *automatically exempted from paying prescription, dental or optical charges; children at school are allowed free meals and children under 5 years and expectant mothers, free welfare milk and foods.*

(c) Supplementary benefits

These are payable as of right to people in Great Britain who are *not* in full-time work and whose other income, whether from other benefits or from their own financial resources, is not enough to meet their requirements. These benefits, therefore, supplement other sources of income.

Supplementary benefits are divided into two types:

(a) *Supplementary pension* for persons over minimum pension age—60 for women, 65 for men.

(b) Supplementary allowance for persons aged 16 and over but under pension age.

The calculation of supplementary benefits is complicated because it depends on the person's resources and requirements. *Certain income resources are disregarded—the first £4 of part-time earnings plus the first £4 of a wife's earnings,* plus £4 of any other regular income. The disregard for one parent families is £4 plus one half of any earnings betwen £4 and £20 weekly. Any attendance or mobility allowance is disregarded.

If a man or his wife own a house they live in, its value is ignored. If a man and his wife have between them capital of *more than £3000 (1983) (including redundency payments) supplementary benefit cannot be obtained.*

Minimum allowances are laid down as indicated in Table 18.1. Discretionary payments have recently been reduced but 'once and for all' payments are still obtainable in emergencies (i.e. fire and flood). Enquiry should be made to the local social security office or from leaflets S.B8, S.B.9, O.C.2.

It is *most important for the nurse to realize that many elderly persons without private means will qualify for special supplementary benefits for rent and extra heating* or *special diet* especially if they are ill or recovering from an illness. *Supplementary benefits are payable as a right* and care

Table 18.1 Supplementary Benefit Table (1983)

	Under pension age	*Over pension age*
Married couple	£43.50	£54.55
Single person (paying rent or owner-occupier)	£26.80	£34.10
Other single person		
* aged 18 or over	£21.45	£27.25
* aged 16–17	£16.50	–

For each dependent child, add to the above rates:

| * aged under 11 | £9.15 | * aged 16–17 | £16.50 |
| * aged 11–15 | £13.70 | * aged 18 or over | £21.45 |

The following can be added, *IF THEY ARE NEEDED* because of age, illness, or other special problems:

* either £2.05, £4.10 or £5.05 (1983) for extra heating
** £3.35 if on a kidney machine, and extra for certain diseases
* cost of laundry if over 40p
* cost of domestic help (but not a local authority home help)

must be taken to point this out because many old people consider that to claim them is in some way degrading and makes them dependent on charity. This is not so and unless old people in need claim, considerable hardship is bound to occur.

Automatic entitlement to other benefits. People and their dependants receiving supplementary benefit are also entitled to exemption from payment of the charges (or to a refund of charges paid) for prescriptions, wigs and fabric supports supplied under the NHS, and NHS dental treatment and certain glasses; children under school age and expectant mothers are also entitled to free milk and vitamins; children at school do not have to pay for school meals; members of the family attending hospital for treatment may claim a refund of fares.

(d) Attendance allowance

This is a tax free allowance for a person who because of his severe physical or mental disabilities requires the following assistance from another person:

By day: frequent attention throughout the day in connection with his bodily functions *or* continual supervision throughout the day in order to avoid substantial danger to himself and others.

At night: prolonged or repeated attention during the night in connection with his bodily functions *or* continual supervision throughout the night in order to avoid substantial danger to himself or others.

In 1983, a higher rate of £27.20 a week can be paid if one of the day requirements *and* one of the night requirements are satisfied for a period of at least 6 months. A lower rate of £18.15 a week can be paid if one of the day *or* night requirements is satisfied for a period of at least six months.

These requirements are strictly enforced and are dealt with by a single Social Security centre in Blackpool. Claims forms are obtainable from any local Social Security office.

(e) Mobility allowance

This new allowance for severely disabled adults has already been described (see page 206). In 1985 it was £20.00 per week.

(f) Non-contributory invalidity pension

This is paid to people of working age who have not been able to work for at least six months *and* who do not have enough national insurance contributions to get invalidity benefit. *Married women can claim only if they are also unable to do normal household work.*

In 1983, it was £20.45 a week (but less if some other benefits are being paid), plus £12.25 for a wife or adult dependant and £7.60 for each child.

(g) Pensions for people over 80

Anyone who is 80 or over and is not receiving a national insurance retirement pension or who is receiving a pension of less than £21.50 a week (1985)—£12.85 for a married woman—may qualify for a non-contributory retirement pension. The person *must* be at least 80 years old and at the time of claiming must normally live in the U.K. and have lived there for a period of at least 10 years in the 20 years ending on their 80th birthday or 19 Sept. 1971, whichever is the later.

(h) Guardian's allowances

A guardian's allowance is a payment to a person who takes into his family an orphan child. The age limits are the same as those for the child benefit. Usually both parents must be dead, but the allowance can be paid on the death of one parent where the parents were divorced; or where the child is illegitimate or where the surviving parent is serving a long term of imprisonment.

One of the child's parents must have been a British subject who was born in the United Kingdom. If neither parent satisfies this condition, one of them must have satisfied a special residence test.

A guardian's allowance *should be claimed not later than three months after a child has joined the family.*

Child benefits are not payable in addition to guardian's allowance.

In 1985 the guardian's allowance was £7.65 a week.

(i) Various industrial injury benefits

Injury and disablement benefits. Payment to persons injured at work or who contract an industrial disease and who are subsequently unable to work is covered by two main benefits:

(a) *Industrial injury benefit* covering the first six months after the injury.

(b) *Industrial disablement pension* or gratuity for any permanent disability after six months.

(a) **Industrial injury benefit** is payable during incapacity for work for the first 26 weeks from the date of accident or industrial disease (usually excludes the first three days). After 26 weeks, anyone still unable to work can get invalidity benefit. Injury benefit is claimed in the same way as sickness benefit.

Industrial injury benefit for those over 18 years of age in 1983 was £27.75 per week with increases for dependent adults and children.

Note: Injury benefit is *not* paid for pneumoconiosis or byssinosis; for both these diseases, disablement benefit can be paid from the start and sickness or invalidity benefit can be paid in addition for anyone unable to work.

(b) **Industrial disablement benefit**. The amount of disablement benefit depends on the extent of disablement as assessed by a medical board.

Disablement of 20 per cent to 100 per cent is taken as qualifying the individual for a disability pension which, in 1983, varied from £55.60 per week for 100 per cent disablement to £10.72 per week for 20 per cent disablement for adults over 18 years of age. For disablement under 19 per cent and under, benefit is usually paid as a disablement gratuity. Up to £3 560 for 19 per cent.

Disablement benefit can also be increased for various additional problems or reasons in the following ways:

Note: All amounts given are those in 1983.

Special hardship allowance. Up to £22.24 a week, as long as the benefit and allowance together do not come to more than £55.60 a week; if as a result of the injury or disease the claimant is unable to return to his regular job or cannot work at a similar job.

Unemployment supplement is paid at £32.60 a week with increases for dependants (at invalidity benefit rates) for anyone who is permanently unfit for work as a result of injury or disease.

Constant attendance allowance is paid of up to £22.30 per week for any one who needs someone to look after him and whose disablement is 100 per cent. In quite exceptional cases, this allowance can be increased to a maximum of £43.00.

Exceptionally severe disablement allowance of £22.30 a week is payable to anyone who is in receipt of constant attendance allowance.

Hospital treatment allowance. This raises the benefit payable to 100 per cent rate, while the claimant is in hospital and receiving treatment for the injury or disease.
Note: For anyone who is incapable of working, sickness benefit or invalidly benefit can be paid in addition to disablement benefit unless an unemployability supplement is also being paid.

Industrial death benefit. Widows and other dependants of an employee who dies as a result of an accident at work or an industrial disease qualify.

For a widow who lived with, or was maintained by, her husband the benefit is £47.65 a week for the first 26 weeks, plus any earnings-related addition. Then £34.60 or £10.22 depending on circumstances. For children of the dead person £7.60 a week is paid with a widow's pension or 15p if paid to some other person.

Invalid Care Allowance is payable to people of working age (16 to 60 for women or 65 for men) who cannot work because they have to stay at home to care for a severely disabled relative (i.e. someone in receipt of either an attendance allowance or a constant attendance allowance).

This benefit is taxable, but it is not means-tested. The person claiming benefit must live in this country and be:

1 regularly and substantially engaged in caring for a severely disabled relative for at least 35 hours per week;
2 not gainfully employed (i.e. any part earnings must not exceed £6 weekly); and
3 not undergoing full-time education.

The rate of allowance is £20.45 per week and normally cannot be backdated for more than 3 months plus £12.25 for a wife or dependent adult and £7.60 for each child.

(j) Employment rehabilitation allowance

This is paid to people who are sick, disabled or unemployed and who are taking a rehabilitation course to help return to work.

In 1983, the amount paid was £36.70 aged over 20 or over and living at home, and smaller amounts for those aged 20 or over and who have to live away from home while on a course, plus earnings related supplement, and for a wife or husband or housekeeper, and for each child.

Claims should be made at the employment office or Job Centre.

(k) Criminal injuries compensation

People covered include those injured as a result of a crime of violence where helping the police or trying to prevent crime or arrest a suspected criminal. It also covers dependants of those killed as a result of a violent crime and victims of violence (if injured after 1st October, 1979).

The benefit is financial compensation based on common law damages dependant upon the amount of pain or suffering caused by the injury and on any loss of earnings or out-of-pocket expenses, subject to a lower compensation level.

If death follows, compensation is assessed in accordance with the Fatal Accidents Act.

Contributory benefits

There are nine contributory benefits:

1   maternity benefits
2   sickness benefits
3   earnings-related supplement
4   invalidity benefit
5   unemployment benefit
6   widows' benefits
7   retirement pensions plus Christmas bonus
8   children's special allowance
9   death grant

(1) Maternity benefits

There are two maternity benefits:

Maternity grant (in 1983, £25.95 for each baby) which is *payable to all insured persons*. It is intended to be a contribution towards the general expense of a confinement. *Maternity allowance* is *payable to women who have paid (or been credited with) full rate National Insurance contribution during the tax year on which their claim is based*. It is usually payable for 18 weeks starting 11 weeks before the baby is expected. It cannot, however, be paid while the woman is working.

In 1983, the maternity allowance was £25.95 a week for up to 18 weeks. In certain circumstances where the woman has dependants, it may be increased in amount.

Claim *must* be made on forms obtainable from local offices of Social Security for *maternity allowance between 14th and 11th week before confinement* and *from 9 weeks before and 3 months after confinement for maternity grant*. Benefit may be lost if a claim is delayed.

Paid maternity leave. A woman who has worked for the same employer for two years or more before the beginning of the 11th week before the baby is due and remains in that job until the beginning of the 11th week, can qualify for paid maternity leave if she stops work to have the baby.

The rate of benefit is 9/10ths of normal weekly pay less the flat rate maternity allowance (see above) whether or not entitled to it. It is paid for first six weeks away from work and is paid by the employer who can claim it back from the Department of Employment.

(2) Sickness benefit

Anyone normally employed or self-employed can claim sickness benefit for the first 28 weeks of any sickness (it is then replaced by invalidity pension—see below). Anyone who falls sick and is incapable of work should obtain from his doctor a medical certificate the first time he sees him. The certificate must be completed (making certain that full details of any dependants, e.g., wife, children are included) and returned to the Social Security office within six days of falling sick.

In 1983, the standard weekly flat-rate sickness benefit for a man or woman (except a married woman) over 18 years of age was £25.95 a week plus earnings related supplement with increases of £16.00 for an adult dependant (including wife) and 15p for each child.

Flat-rate sickness benefit is not paid for the first three days of any spell of sickness or for isolated days of illness.

N.B. From April 1983 the government proposes that, instead of sickness benefit, employees will get a statutory minimum of sick pay from employers for the first 8 weeks in any year.

(3) Earnings related supplement

People receiving sickness benefit, injury benefit, unemployment benefit, maternity allowance (after second week) widow's allowance, TOPs training allowance or employment rehabilitation allowance may qualify for an *earnings-related supplement*. The amount depends on what was earned during the previous year. The most payable is £14 a week (if Class 1 contributions have been paid on earnings of £6750 a year or more). For sickness, injury, unemployment or maternity benefit the total (basic and extra for dependants and supplement) cannot exceed 85 per cent of earnings on which the supplement is based.

(4) Invalidity benefit

This normally replaces sickness benefit after 28 weeks of illness.

Invalidity pension replaces sickness benefit in all cases and *invalidity allowance* is added as an extra weekly payment to people who become chronically sick while they still have a large part of their normal working lives ahead of them.

In 1985, the invalidity pension was £34.25 a week with increases of £20.55 for an adult dependant. The wife of a man drawing invalidity pension can earn £35.00 a week before the increase paid for her is affected provided she resides with him.

Invalidity allowance depends on the age of incapacity—the earlier the incapacity the larger the allowance. In 1985 it varied from £7.50 a week for those whose incapacity started under the age of 40 years to £4.80 per week for those whose incapacity started after 40 years of age but before 50 years and £2.40 if at least 50 but under 60 (men) or under 55 (women). *Note*: Earnings-related supplement (see below) is *not* payable with invalidity benefit.

(5) Unemployment benefit

This is paid only while a person in unemployed, capable of work and available to take a job.

Unemployment benefit in 1983 was £27.05 with increases of £16.70 for an adult dependent. It is payable for up to 312 days in any period of interruption of employment. Once benefit has run out, unemployment benefit cannot be paid until the claimant has been back at work and paid 13 Class 1 flat-rate contributions.

On the first day of unemployment, the claimant should register for work at an Employment Exchange and claim benefit. If under 18 years of age, he should attend the Careers Office (Youth Employment Office) if there is one in the district or a Job Centre.

(6) Redundancy payments

Those who have worked for at least 2 years continuously for an employer and are under 65 (man) or 60 (woman) and who are made redundant from their job qualify for redundancy payments. This is a tax free lump sum of at least:

1    $1\frac{1}{2}$ weeks pay for each year's service between 41 and retirement age, plus
2   1 weeks pay for each year's service between 22 and 41, plus
3    $\frac{1}{2}$ week's pay for each year's service between 18 and 22.

20 years service is the most that can count and the highest weekly pay on which the lump sum is worked out is £135 (1983). These are minimum figures and can be increased by agreement.

(7) Widow's benefits

There are two main types of widows' benefits. All widows, whose husbands' contributions are sufficient, qualify for a **widows' allowance** payable for six months. After this period, benefit is only given to widows with dependent children (**widowed mothers' allowance**) and to widows over 40 years of age (**widows' pension**).

Widows' allowance in 1985 was £50.10 a week (payable for the first 26 weeks of widowhood) with increases for dependent children of £7.65 for each child and usually an earnings related supplement (see page 279).

If a woman is widowed when aged 60 years or over, she can get the allowance only if her husband was not a pensioner.

Widowed mothers' allowance. After six months, a widow with a dependent child or who is expecting a child by her late husband will get a widowed mothers' allowance. The basic allowance in 1985 was £35.80 a week with similar increases for children as with widows' allowance (see above).

(If the children have left school and are under 19 years of age and still living with the widow, she can get a smaller allowance without additions for children.)

Widows' pension is paid to two main groups:

(a) to a widow if she does not qualify at the termination of her widow's allowance for a widowed mothers' allowance, and was over the age of 40 years when her husband died; *or*

(b) a widow after she ceases to be entitled to a widowed mothers' allowance if she is then over the age of 40 years.

In 1985, the standard rate for a widow's pension was £35.80 a week if she was over 50 when her husband died or when her widowed mother's allowance ended. Below the age of 50, the widow's pension ranges from £10.74 for a childless widow under 40 to £35.80 at 50.

Widow's benefits cease if the widow remarries or cohabits with a man as his wife. All widows over 60 can get a retirement pension of at least as much as the widow's pension they were receiving before they left work.

(8) Retirement pension

At 65 (60 for a woman) an individual who retires from regular work and satisfies the contribution conditions can get a retirement pension.

When a man reaches 70 (a woman 65) a pension is payable whether retired or not.

In 1985, the amount payable for retirement pensions is made up of:

(a) *Basic retirement pension* of £35.80 a week.

(b) Increases of £21.50 a week for a wife who is not entitled to a pension herself.

Extra pension can be earned by deferring retirement beyond 65 (60 for women).

Graduated pension may also be added in respect of any graduated contributions paid between 1961 and 1975 (when graduated contributions ceased).

Age addition of 25 pence is payable to all pensioners aged 80 or over.

The earnings rule. If a man is under 70 and a woman under 65, and does paid work after retirement, the retirement pension is reduced by 5 p

(i) for every 10 p earned between £70 and £74 a week (1985);
(ii) for each 5 p earned over £74 a week.

(9) Children's special allowance

This is an allowance to a woman whose marriage has been dissolved or annulled if, on the death of a former husband, she has a child towards whose support he was contributing (or had been liable to do so) at least 25 p a week. In 1983, the allowance was £7.60 for each child. Child Benefit is, of course, payable in addition (see page 274). This allowance cannot be paid if the woman has remarried.

(10) Death grant

A death grant is a sum payable to the next of kin, executor or person paying the funeral expenses on the death of an insured person or of the wife, husband or child of an insured person. It can also be paid on the contributions of a close relative in respect of a handicapped person who has never been able to work.

If the deceased person left a will, the grant is paid to the executors; otherwise it is paid to the person meeting the funeral expenses.

The amount varies with age. In 1985 it varied between £9 and £30 depending on the age of the dead person.

Entitlements to certain services at no cost or at reduced cost if the individual qualifies

There is a general entitlement to certain services at no cost or at a reduced cost if the person qualifies in a special group. Examples include:

At no cost:
Prescription charges
Dental charges
Charges for optical glasses
Hospital travel fares
Free school meals
Milk and vitamins
At reduced cost:
Legal advice and assistance
Rent rebates
Rate rebates

Prescription charges

Medicines and appliances prescribed under the National Health Service are supplied free to the following persons on completion of the declaration on the back of the prescription form:

Children under 16.
Men aged 65 or over and women aged 60 or over.
Holders of exemption certificates:
    Expectant and nursing mothers (i.e. mothers who have a child under 1 year old);
    People suffering from certain medical conditions;
    War or service disablement pensioners (for prescriptions required for their accepted disablements);

People or their dependants receiving supplementary benefit or family income supplement.

In addition, anyone who is not covered by the above exemptions, but whose income is below a certain level is entitled to exemption.

If anyone does not qualify but needs prescriptions frequently, it is possible to buy a prescription 'season ticket' covering all NHS prescription charges for either four months or 12 months.

Dental charges

The following persons are exempt from dental charges:

1   All children under 16.
2   Young people aged 16 and over who are still attending school.
3   For all those aged 16 and 17, and for those aged 18 who are in full-time education (either at school or elsewhere). Dentures are free to those aged 16–18 who are in full time education.
4   Expectant mothers.
5   Women who have had a child within the previous 12 months.
6   Persons and their dependants who are receiving supplementary pension or allowance.
7   Persons in a family receiving family income supplement.
8   Persons, and their dependants, who are exempt from prescription charges *on income grounds*.
9   Persons in a family receiving milk and vitamins free *on income grounds*.

To claim exemption the patient will be asked to sign a declaration on the dentist's treatment form. Hospital *in-patients* are not charged for dental treatment or dentures.

Charges for National Health Service (NHS) glasses

The following qualify automatically for free NHS glasses:

1   those on supplementary benefit;
2   persons in a family receiving family income supplement;
3   people already getting free milk or prescriptions *because of low income*;
4   children under 16;
5   young people over 16 still at school.

It may be possible to get help if the individual has no automatic right, but has not much money coming in.

Free National Health Service (NHS) hearing aid

People of all ages with impaired hearing for whom a hearing aid is prescribed by a consultant can get the NHS aid supplied and fitted, serviced, maintained and supplied with batteries free of charge from the special hearing aid centre attached to certain hospitals.

Initially reference must be by a family doctor.

How a stay in hospital affects social security benefits

A number of social security benefits are affected on admission to hospital either immediately or after a short period. The following is an indication, but enquiry must be made to the local social security office, who should be told of any admission.

(a) *On immediate admission* of claimant or dependant—supplementary benefit may be affected at once;

(b) *After four weeks in hospital* attendance allowance and constant attendance allowance;

(c) *After eight weeks in hospital* Sickness or invalidity benefit, non-contributory invalidity pension, widow's benefits, retirement pension, injury benefit, industrial widow's or widower's pensions and unemploy-ability supplements;

(d) After 52 weeks—war widow's pension;

(e) the invalid care allowance time limit differs according to circumstances.

There is no need to notify the social security office if the hospital stay is less than these limits or if the individual is being treated as an out-patient (even with odd days in hospital).

Hospital fares

Patients. Hospital patients who are receiving supplementary benefit or family income supplement can have their fares to and from hospital refunded on production of their order book when they attend for treatment. Patients not receiving supplementary benefit may also be entitled to help with their fares, if there is not much money coming into the household. The fares of a person accompanying a patient to hospital may also be paid if his presence on the journey is medically necessary. War pensioners can claim if they attend hospital for treatment (as in-patients or out-patients) for their pensionable disablement. Relatives may also claim if they visit war pensioners in hospital. The hospital social worker will advise how to claim.

Free school meals

Free school meals are available for schoolchildren in families receiving supplementary benefit, family income supplement or are in special need because of low income. Enquiry at school or at the local Education Office will indicate the steps which any parent must take to obtain this help.

Milk and vitamins

Liquid milk (7 pints per week) or its equivalent in dried milk, Vitamin A, D, and C drops for children (2 bottles every 13 weeks) and Vitamin A, D and C tablets for mothers (expectant mothers 2 containers every 13 weeks; nursing mothers 5 containers in all) are available free of charge for an expectant mother and all children including foster children under school age in families who are receiving supplementary benefits, family income supplement or are in special need because of low income.

Free milk is also available for:

(a) Handicapped children aged 5 to 15 who are not registered pupils at a special school or ordinary school (7 pints per week).

(b) Children attending an approved day nursery or play group or with an approved child minder ($\frac{1}{3}$ pint each day they attend). A few local education authorities provide free school milk.

Any mother wishing to claim milk etc. should contact her local health visitor or child health clinic.

Legal advice and assistance

People of small or moderate means and few savings may obtain legal advice and assistance for little or no payment from a solicitor, as if they were fee-paying clients, on any subject usually dealt with by a solicitor. This includes giving advice, writing letters, drafting wills, obtaining opinions from a barrister, preparing a written statement to help someone who has to appear before an administrative or appeal tribunal and visiting a police station or prison.

This help does not extend to representation in proceedings before a court or tribunal but, if representation is needed for proceedings in court, either civil or criminal, the solicitor will advise his client how to apply for legal aid. Legal aid is not generally available for proceedings before tribunals.

Information as to how to apply for legal advice and assistance is available from Citizens' Advice Bureaux, public libraries or by post from The Law Society, 113 Chancery Lane, London WC21 1PL or from The Law Society of Scotland, 27 Drumsheugh Gardens, Edinburgh EH3 7YR.

Rent rebates and allowances

Most tenants who find it difficult to afford the full rent (*except those already receiving supplementary benefit*, because this includes an element for rent) may apply to their local authority for direct financial help. Local authority tenants who qualify receive a rent rebate which is deducted at source from their rents.

The amount of rebate or allowance is governed by three main factors, the tenant's gross income (including his wife's), the size of his family, and his rent (excluding rates and services).

People who are having difficulty in paying their rent should seek information from Citizens' Advice Bureaux or their Local Authority.

Rate rebates

Owner-occupiers and tenants (including those who pay rates as part of their rent) who are not receiving supplementary benefit can claim a rebate on their general rates from a local authority. Residents of commercial or mixed properties can qualify for a rebate on the domestic part.

Many old people, may qualify (see page 249). Anyone who is *in doubt whether he qualifies should always apply*. All applications are treated in the strictest confidence. Application forms and further details of the scheme can be obtained from the local council.

Index